The Practical Dash Diet

Maple Grove Press

The Practical Dash Diet

© Copyright 2018 by Maple Grove Press - All rights reserved.

Contents

Introduction	5
Overview	7
What is DASH Diet?	7
The History of DASH Diet	7
How does the DASH Diet work?	7
Benefits of the DASH Diet	8
Best Foods to Eat on the DASH Diet	9
Foods You'll Want to Limit on the DASH Diet	16
Make Gradual Changes	23
Limit Meat Consumption	23
Substitute Healthy Desserts	24
Reduce Oils	24
Increase Your Dairy Intake	25
I. The Positive Impact of Dash Diet	26
1.) A Wholesome Diet – Dash Diet	26
2.) Take Control of Your Blood Pressure	26
3.) The NEW Added Benefit of the Dash Diet –Cholesterol Management	27
4.) The Weight Management Plan	27
II. The Complexities of the Dash Diet	27
1.) Taste Issues –Where's the SALT?	28
2.) Calorie Check – The Ups and Downs	28
DASH Diet FAQ	29
Is the DASH diet only for hypertension?	29
Does it follow a phase system?	29
Is it good for losing weight?	29
Is the DASH diet for all ages?	29
Is it ideal for busy professionals?	30
Are the results fast?	30

Are the results noticeable?	30
Is it suitable for vegetarians?	30
Is it sustainable?	30

DASH Tips for Busy People — 31

Stock up on nutritional snacks	31
Stick to your list	31
Befriend your refrigerator	31
Be creative in transforming leftovers	32
Hydrate	32
Fitness	32
Other lifestyle choices	34
Positive actions	34
Why the DASH diet is sustainable	35

Dash Kitchen: — 36

Essential Equipment	36
Nice-to-Have Equipment	37

Eating Out on the Dash Diet: — 40

Dash Diet for Weight Loss — 40

Keep a Food Journal	40
Calculate Your Calorie Goal	40

Phase 1: Shed Weight Two Weeks — 41

Phase 2: Kick It Up a Notch! — 41

Make the Transition Slowly	42
Reduce Your Consumption of Fat and Sugar Even Further	42
Limit Sodium to 1,500 mg per Day	42
Eat More Vegetables and Whole Grains	42
Fat-Free is Not Always Healthy	43
Distribute Your Calories Throughout the Day	43
Exercise Plan	43
Interval Training	44
Weight Training is the King of All Weight-Loss Workouts	45
Running	45
Train Like a Boxer	45
Jumping Rope	46

The Practical Dash Diet

Making DASH Work For You:	47
Are You Trying Losing Weight or Manage Your Blood Pressure?	47
The BMR	47
Getting Started with The DASH Diet	49
Some Words on Sodium	49
Dash Recipe Box:	51
Easy Veggie Muffins	51
Carrot Muffins	52
Pineapple Oatmeal	53
Spinach Muffins	54
Chia Seeds Breakfast Mix	56
Breakfast Fruits Bowls	57
Pumpkin Breakfast Cookies	58
Delicious Veggie Quesadillas	59
Chicken Wraps	60
Black Bean Patties	62
Lunch Rice Bowls	63
Salmon Sandwich	64
Stuffed Mushrooms Caps	66
Lunch Tuna Salad	67
Oven Roasted Herbed Carrots	68
Tasty Grilled Asparagus	69
Easy Roasted Broccoli	71
Baked Potato Mix	72
Spicy Brussels Sprouts	73
Easy Slow Cooked Potatoes	75
Squash Side Salad	76
Colored Iceberg Salad	77
Chicken Parmesan:	78
Slow Cooker Turkey Sweet Potato Chili:	80
Fennel Side Salad	82
Shrimp Salad with Grilled Peaches:	83
Corn Mix	84
Mediterranean Chicken with Quinoa	85
Persimmon Side Salad	87
14 Day Dash Meal Plan:	89

Shopping Lists	100
DASH Shopping List	101
How to Read Labels	104
Using the Numbers from Labels and Food Lists	105
Conclusion	106

Introduction

It's the 21st century and we've made great advances in things like technology and medicine. However, when it comes to our personal health, we seem to have taken a step back. People today are ridden with things like Type 2 Diabetes and cardiovascular disease among other things. Obesity is a constant problem. Why is it that we've made such great improvements in certain areas like technology, yet the obesity rate continues to increase?

It comes down to the wrong information. We are constantly being sold on gimmicks like weight loss pills and other sketchy powders and potions that are supposed to magically help us lose weight, get our blood pressure in check, and make us healthy again. But clearly none of those things are working. We try diet after diet in the hopes that it'll finally be the answer, and all we end up with is disappointment.

Luckily this all changes for you today. In this book, you'll discover what has been named as the best diet multiple years in a row by countless scientific journals, medical professionals and (most importantly) regular people like you and me. It's not some gimmicky overnight fix. Instead it's something that actually works on a biological and physiological level helping you to actually heal your body and improve your health—not just treat the symptoms.

I'm talking about the DASH diet here. This nutritional approach will finally allow you to lose weight and get your health back on track. Not only that, but it isn't that hard of a diet to follow! Most diets have confusing rules like you can only eat at a certain time or they force you to eat certain foods.

That won't be the case with the DASH diet. In this book, you'll learn about all of the ins and outs of the DASH lifestyle. You'll understand all of the health benefits you can expect to gain from following this eating plan. You'll even learn how to use exercise to further benefit your nutrition plan. And finally, you'll be given a step-by-step process along with a 14-day sample meal plan to help you get started on the right foot with the DASH diet. Let's dive in and get started...

Overview

What is DASH Diet?

The word DASH comes from the acronym Dietary Approaches to Stop Hypertension. In the year 1992, the National Heart, Lung and Blood Institute (NHLBI) conducted a research study seeking ways to reduce critical blood pressure and cardiovascular health problems in the United States. The DASH study involved doctors, nutritionists and other medical representatives from the top 5 health Centre's of US.

The original research resulted in forming a wholesome nutrition plan known as Dash Diet that helped people in reducing their high blood pressure (or hypertension).

Researchers from various institutes concluded that the Dash diet was one of the best plans to adopt if you have one of the four problems,

1.)   Blood Pressure
2.)   Cholesterol
3.)   Diabetes
4.)   Weight issues

The History of DASH Diet

Due to the rising number of people that are overweight and obese and who struggle with other related diseases, the National Institute of Health together with other organizations across the United Sates conducted a comprehensive research study on these threatening diseases. The outcome showed that the eating habits of individuals is the single most important factor that effects their weight and unhealthy weight gain leads to hypertension. Because of this situation, the DASH Diet or Dietary Approaches to Stop Hypertension was formulated. The DASH Diet intends to lower blood pressure without any aid of medication; it is an all-natural plan that has become an established model of healthy eating.

How does the DASH Diet work?

The food plan focuses on fruits, vegetables, non-fat/low-fat dairy and whole grains such as cereals. The eating plan also includes the consumption of high fiber foods, medium to low amounts of fat, low red meat, and less sugar. An additional benefit of this diet is that it is rich in different vitamins and minerals that are important in achieving a healthy body.

Another good thing about this diet plan is that it lowers your sodium intake in your diet (daily consumption for sodium is only 2,3oo mg on the dash diet) that will help regulate blood pressure levels. That's because studies show that eating food with high sodium content could lead to a spike in blood pressure.

The diet plan has claimed to lower the blood pressure in just two weeks and has

The Practical Dash Diet

been recommended by Centers for Disease Control, American Heart Association, The National Heart, Lung, and Blood Institute, the Mayo Clinic, US Government guidelines for treatment of high blood pressure and a lot more.

Benefits of the DASH Diet

Aside from lowering blood pressure and helping you lose weight, several studies also claim that it can prevent other diseases such as cancer, stroke, heart failure, diabetes, kidney stones, and osteoporosis.

For diabetes, the high-fiber food consumption that is part of the DASH Diet (minimum intake is about 30g of fiber daily) does not only help promote better digestive health, but it can also control glucose and insulin production; which also makes it a great food plan for diabetics.

The other advantages of the DASH diet are: reversing ageing effects, strengthening the bones, joints and muscles, rejuvenating the hair and skin, reducing cholesterol levels, cutting the risk factor of metabolic syndrome, and improving heart health. Exercise or regular workouts are recommended with the DASH Diet in order to reap further health benefits.

Remember, this diet is not just any fad diet. This is not the type of diet where: once you achieved your health/weight goals in "x" amount of time, you will quit the diet. The point of the diet is an overall lifestyle change to be maintained for a healthier you.

Anyone who makes a change to their diet will experience the symptoms of that change. The experience will be different for everyone because people come to the DASH diet from unique starting points in terms of diet quality and composition. However, knowing that your mind and body need to adjust to change will help you keep moving forward.

What to Expect in the Short Term:

If you are used to following a more standard American diet, you may find that your transition to the DASH eating plan will result in unexpected side effects, both positive and negative ones. Drastically reducing the amount of salt, fat, sugar, and refined carbohydrates could lead to cravings for the foods you initially cut from your diet.

Remember, these cravings are only temporary, and once your body gets used to a lower intake, your palate will change and you will no longer experience cravings. Be prepared for when cravings strike and keep your kitchen stocked with healthy snacks like fresh fruits and vegetables. On the positive side, cutting out sources of empty calories will surely lead to a welcome loss of weight, especially if you combine the DASH diet with a regular exercise program.

What to Expect in the Long Term

Depending on how closely you follow the DASH eating pattern, you may find your blood-pressure readings decrease by several points in just two weeks. In the long term, following the DASH diet will reduce your risk of cancer, lower your risk for metabolic syndrome, lower your risk for type 2 diabetes, decrease your heart-disease risk, and, if you are overweight, help you shed the pounds. You may also find you sleep better, your digestion could improve, and you could experience more energy.

Best Foods to Eat on the DASH Diet

The following are the best foods you can eat while on the DASH diet. These are foods that are high in fiber, magnesium, potassium, and other vitamins and minerals. This is not meant to be a comprehensive list, rather this is meant to give you some good ideas for what you should be eating while on the DASH diet.

Vegetables

While following the DASH diet, you should be consuming around 4-5 servings of vegetables per day. We all know that vegetables are good for us and that they are very healthy foods, yet I think few of us realize just how healthy vegetables really are:

➢ Eating vegetables regularly can help to reduce the risk of heart disease and stroke (5).

➢ It can help protect you against certain types of cancer (6).

➢ Vegetables are low in calories and high in fiber. This means that you can eat as many of them as you want and not have to worry about overeating. And the fiber will help to keep you fuller for a longer period of time as well as ensure proper bowel movements. (this generally applies to non-starchy vegetables. Vegetables like corn and potatoes should generally be eaten in moderation since they are higher in calories and carbohydrates.)

➢ Vegetables are very nutrient dense, meaning that they contain a lot of nutrients even though they're low in overall calories. Something like a candy bar, on the other hand, isn't nutrient dense. It contains a lot of calories, but it has very few nutrients.

➢ Folic acid: folic acid helps the body to create red blood cells. Red blood cells are necessary for transporting oxygen throughout your body. Getting proper amounts of folic acid is especially important for pregnant women or women who plan on becoming pregnant to ensure proper fetal development.

➢ Vegetables are rich in so many vitamins and minerals! Vegetables contain high amounts of vitamin A, C, potassium, iron, magnesium, and calcium.

➢ Vegetables are delicious. Very few foods are as versatile in how you can prepare them. If you think vegetables taste boring, you're doing it wrong. There are so many ways you can dress your vegetables up and make them taste shockingly delicious.

Here's a list of vegetables that you should consume on the DASH diet:

➢ Sweet potatoes
➢ Tomatoes

> Squash
> Spinach
> Potatoes
> Lima Beans
> Kale
> Green Beans
> Peas
> Collard Greens
> Mustard Greens
> Broccoli
> Cauliflower
> Carrots

Fruits

Just like vegetables, fruits are very good for you and will provide you with many of the same vitamins and minerals that vegetables will. Unfortunately, fruits sometimes get a bad reputation because they contain fructose, which is a type of sugar. The thing is though that fructose is a natural sugar, not a processed sugar, and the benefits you'll receive from eating fruits far outweighs the fact that they contain some sugar in them.

While following the DASH diet eating plan, you'll want to consume 4-5 servings of fruit per day. Here are some of the amazing benefits of eating fruit:

> Fruits contain low amounts of sodium, calories, and fat.

> Similar to vegetables, fruit is very nutrient dense. So basically, you'll be getting a good bang-for-your-buck when it comes to getting the most nutrients for the least amount of calories. Eating rich nutrient dense foods is critical for your success with the DASH diet.

> Fruits can help to lower cholesterol levels as well as reduce the risk for heart disease (7).

> Additionally, fruits contain high amounts of vitamin A and C, potassium, magnesium, folic acid, and fiber.

> Fruits also contain high amounts of water, which will help to keep your body hydrated.

> Some fruits and especially berries are seen as "superfoods" for their antioxidant properties. Consumption of these fruits have been linked to reduction in risks for certain cancers and other types of diseases.

Here's a list of fruits you should consume on the DASH diet:

> Raisins
> Blueberries
> Raspberries

The Practical Dash Diet

- ➢ Strawberries
- ➢ Peaches
- ➢ Pineapples
- ➢ Melons
- ➢ Grapes
- ➢ Apples
- ➢ Apricots
- ➢ Bananas
- ➢ Dates
- ➢ Oranges
- ➢ Grapefruit
- ➢ Mangoes
- ➢ Tangerines

Dairy

While on the DASH diet eating plan, you should be consuming around 2-3 servings of dairy per day. It's important to note that you'll want to be eating low-fat dairy. The DASH diet limits certain types of fat intake, and consuming large amounts of fat through dairy isn't ideal, especially if it can be avoided in the first place. Here are some of the key benefits of consuming dairy in your diet:

➢ Dairy is high in protein. Protein is one of three macronutrients (carbs and fat being the other two), and it's responsible for aiding in many of your body's functions. One of the main things protein does is rebuild and repair tissue.

➢ It's an important building block for muscle, bone, skin, cartilage, and blood. It's also needed for the growth of hair and nails. So needless to say, protein is a very critical nutrient regardless if you're looking to pack on muscle or not.

➢ Dairy is rich in calcium. When you think of strong bones, what do you think of? You probably think of some kid or adult drinking a glass of milk. We've really been bombarded with the fact that milk (and other dairy products for that matter) is good for strong bones, and it really is so true! This is all because of calcium. Calcium is necessary for maintaining bone mass in the body, which helps to support the skeleton.

The thing is though we lose a lot of calcium through normal bodily processes in the kidneys and colon. Calcium is also used in muscle and nerve functions as well. And if we don't supply our bodies with enough calcium, then our bodies will start to pull the stored calcium in our bones in order to carry out its normal everyday functions.

This is why it's so important to be able to get the proper amount of calcium. It's not just used for our bones, but for many other necessary functions of our bodies. If we're not consuming an adequate amount of calcium, then that's when our bones will take a hit.

The Practical Dash Diet

They'll start to become more brittle and frail. This can then lead to osteoporosis. Approximately 44 million Americans suffer from osteoporosis or low bone mass, and 55% of Americans over the age of 50 have osteoporosis (8). Osteoporosis will lead to more bone and hip fractures, which will inhibit mobility along with making it much harder to follow a diet plan such as DASH.

The following are some good sources of dairy that you can eat. Remember to go with the low-fat option when possible:

- Skim Milk
- 1% Milk
- Low-Fat Cheese
- Low-Fat Cottage Cheese
- Low-Fat Yogurt

This is one of the many differentiators of the DASH diet vs. other diets. One of the biggest issues with so many other diets out there is that there's a calcium deficiency. Medical professionals are always criticizing the leading diets for this. In the short-term it may not cause many problems, but long term it can lead to pre-mature aging, bone deterioration and other diseases. With the DASH diet, you won't have to worry about that. You'll probably even be consuming more calcium than you previously were. This is one of the things I really love about the DASH diet. It's so balanced. It's not trying to just focus on one thing—it helps you improve your health holistically with minimal side effects.

Meats, Poultry, and Fish

You'll also be consuming some meat on the DASH diet plan. Meat isn't as heavily emphasized as some of the other food groups, such as fruits and vegetables however, it's still an important part of the diet regime. You'll want to consume around 1-2 servings of meat, poultry, and/or fish per day.

When consuming these meats, you'll want to make sure that you're going with lean meats. Additionally, be sure to trim away any visible fat from the meat that you can. Finally, the way you cook and prepare the meat matters as well. Avoid frying the food as this will make it have excess fat that isn't necessary. Instead, you'll want to broil, roast, or poach the meat.

This is the healthiest way to prepare your food. On a side note, when you're preparing poultry, remove the skin. Getting rid of the skin will help to remove more of the fat content contained in the chicken. Here are some of the benefits of consuming meat, poultry, and fish:

The Practical Dash Diet

- High in protein: Similar to dairy products, any meat that you consume will have a good amount of protein in it. As mentioned earlier, this is important for repairing muscle tissue, growing hair and nails, as well as being an important building block for skin, bone, cartilage, and blood.

- Lean meats also contain a high amount of magnesium. Magnesium is critical for the proper functioning of hundreds of enzymes. Research has shown that magnesium can help to reduce blood pressure with individuals who are suffering from hypertension (9).

It can also help with type 2 diabetes (10). And it can even help to fight depression (11). Fortunately, the DASH diet will allow you to consume plenty of magnesium, not just from lean meats, but from other food sources as well. Here's a list of lean meats that you can consume:

- Poultry
- Fish
- Bison
- Venison
- Beef

Nuts, Seeds, and Dried Beans

You'll want to consume 3 servings of various nuts, seeds, and dried beans per week on the DASH diet. You'll be eating quite a bit less of this food group compared to some of the other food groups, and it's for a good reason. Nuts are comprised mostly of fat.

Yes, there are good types of fat and bad types of fat (more on this later), however fat contains 9 calories per gram. On the other hand, protein and carbs only contain 4 calories per gram of food. This means that you'll be consuming over twice the amount of calories for the same amount of food if you're consuming fat. Those calories can add up rather quickly, and this is something we want to be aware of.

That's why you'll only be consuming 3 servings per week of these different nuts, seeds, and dried beans. As I just mentioned though, there is such a thing as good fat and bad fat. Bad fats would be something like trans-fat and saturated fat. Excessive amounts of these types of fat have been shown to increase the risk for heart disease as well as other health problems (12).

Nuts and seeds, on the other hand, contain mono and polyunsaturated fats. These are a healthy type of fat that can help to lower your risk of heart disease by decreasing your low-density lipoproteins (LDL) and maintaining your high-density lipoproteins (HDL). Your LDL's are the bad type of cholesterol, and your HDL's are the good kind of cholesterol.

The Practical Dash Diet

Of course, this idea of there being a good type of fat might be hard for you to grasp at first. Just like myself, you probably grew up learning that fat is bad for you. Intuitively this makes sense because we can see how excess fat on our bodies is bad for us so it naturally makes sense that consuming fat is harmful. However, this couldn't be further from the truth.

The reality is that consuming too many calories overall from all three macronutrients (protein, carbs, and fat) is bad for us and that's what leads to weight gain. Yes, certain types of fat should be limited or avoided altogether (such as saturated or trans-fat), but that's not to say that all fat is bad for you because that simply isn't the case. Here are some of the benefits of consuming nuts, seeds, and dried beans:

- They are a rich source of energy. As I talked about earlier, fat contains 9 calories per gram. This can be dangerous if overeaten, however you have to remember why we're eating food in the first place—to get energy! Our body needs daily energy to maintain itself and carry out its daily functions.

And where do our bodies get that needed energy? It gets it from the foods that we eat of course! Eating nuts is a great way to give our bodies a solid source of calories if we need to consume more. Just be careful not to overdo it!

- Contain healthy amounts of magnesium and fiber. Are you starting to notice a common theme here? Many of the foods you'll be consuming on the DASH diet are rich in magnesium! It's such a key mineral for getting and staying healthy, especially if you have hypertension.

Not only that, but nuts, seeds, and dried beans contain fiber. This is something that the typical American doesn't get enough of, and it's no wonder why so many people struggle with digestive issues.

- Finally, this food group surprisingly contains a good amount of protein. This is something you might not expect at first, but it's certainly true. For example, one serving of almonds contains 6 grams of protein! So not only will you be consuming healthy fats when you eat nuts, but you'll also be getting a decent amount of protein as well.

Now that you know the benefits of this food group, here's a list of some different kinds of them you can eat on the DASH diet (of course always go with the unsalted version whenever possible):

- Almonds
- Hazelnuts
- Mixed Nuts
- Peanuts

- Walnuts
- Sunflower Seeds
- Natural Peanut Butter
- Natural Almond Butter
- Kidney Beans
- Lentils
- Split Peas

Yes, on many other diets, nuts and beans are a very important part of the diet, and of course we agree that the healthy benefits of these foods are real—in moderation. As with everything on the DASH diet, we want to stick to things that are measurable. The problem with other diets when they say you should eat nuts instead of non-nutritive snacks is that there's not much to help you measure this. If you just go around throwing handfuls of almonds into your mouth, you'll be thinking that you're being healthy, without being aware of the massive amounts of calories you're consuming. This can not only stagnate weight loss, but even contribute to weight gain. Thus, the DASH diet wisely and specifically outlines exactly how much of this food group you can consume so that you can reap the health benefits, without having to deal with the associates issues.

Fats and Oils

Fats and oils are another essential part of the DASH diet. Again, fats have gotten a bad reputation over the years, but it isn't all justified. The same goes for oils. When you think of oily food, what do you typically think of? Probably something that's greasy, fried, contains a lot of fat, and is unhealthy for you right?

Well yes, some oils are really bad for you. However, not all oils are as bad as they might seem. As I mentioned earlier, there are good fats and bad fats. You want to limit bad fats in your diet such as saturated fat and trans-fat.

And you'll want to consume more healthy fats like mono and polyunsaturated fats. That's why you'll want to use oils that contain healthy fats like mono and polyunsaturated fats. The best kind of oil you can use is olive oil. This is a healthy type of oil that contains a good amount of monounsaturated fat.

Canola oil can be a good option to use as well due to its high monounsaturated fat content as well but use olive oil when you can as a first option. In terms of how much fats and oils you should be consuming, try to get roughly 2 servings of fats and oils per day. Here are some of the benefits of consuming fats and oils:

➤ Regulation of body temperature: Fats are important for regulating your body temperature and helping to keep it at a normal and healthy range.

➤ Good for brain health: non-water-soluble vitamins such as vitamins A, D, E, and K need fat to get absorbed and transported by the body. These vitamins are critical for a properly functioning brain. Not only that, but your brain is made up of close to 60% fat (13)! So needless to say, it's quite important that you get an adequate amount of fat in your diet.

> ➤ Source of energy: fat can be stored in the body for later use, however it can also be used as a more primary source of energy if the body is low on carbohydrates or low on calories.

> ➤ Healthy skin and hair: Fat can help to make skin and hair appear soft, silky, and smooth due to its protective qualities. Without this protection from fat, harmful chemicals would be able to more easily enter the body through the skin.

Whole Grains

On the DASH eating plan, you're going to want to consume 6-8 servings of whole grains per day. It's very important to note that you'll want to be consuming *whole grains* here and not refined grains. Refined grains are more processed than whole grains and thus lose vitamins, minerals, and fiber during the process which means you'll basically just be consuming empty calories when consuming refined grains.

Whole grains, on the other hand, contain more vitamins and fiber, which is key to keeping you fuller longer. Whole grains still contain all three parts of the grain, which are the bran, germ, and endosperm.

When refined grains get processed, they're stripped of the bran and germ, which contain many key nutrients. Not only that, but whole grains are rich in things such as thiamin, riboflavin, niacin, and folate. These are part of the B vitamins complex. B vitamins are important for many different things including:

> ➤ Making new cells
> ➤ Red cell production
> ➤ Increase in HDL cholesterol (which is the good kind of cholesterol)
> ➤ Preventing memory loss
> ➤ Keeping depression at bay

Here's a list of acceptable whole grains should you eat while on the DASH diet:

> ➤ Whole-wheat pasta
> ➤ Whole-wheat bread
> ➤ Brown rice
> Whole-grain cereal

Foods You'll Want to Limit on the DASH Diet

One of the things I really like about the DASH diet is that it doesn't entirely forbid you to eat the foods you love. I've seen plenty of people start a new diet plan only to fail a few short weeks later when they couldn't handle the misery anymore. Here's how

The Practical Dash Diet

it usually goes down:

1. You start a new diet and get all excited about it.
2. You immediately go cold turkey and cut all junk food from your diet.
3. For the first few days and maybe even weeks, things go pretty smoothly.
4. Then something comes up, like your best friend's birthday party for example.
5. While at the party, you do your best to stay on track with your diet plan.
6. You see everyone around you having a good time and eating as they please.
7. You really can't handle it anymore so you tell yourself you've been good and one piece of cake can't hurt that bad right?
8. You eat the piece of cake and then proceed to binge eat everything in sight.
9. Later that night you feel guilty for binge eating junk food and feel disgusted with yourself.

10. You also wonder if you'll ever be able to get the hang of this diet thing.

11. Then a few days or weeks later when you're feeling better about yourself, you start a new diet and the cycle repeats itself.

You see the problem in the above scenario isn't the fact that the person ate a slice of birthday cake. The reality is that one piece of cake, one brownie, one bowl of ice cream, etc. can't completely wreck your diet in one fell swoop. What does ruin your diet is when you feel guilty for eating something you feel like you shouldn't have.

These feelings of guilt then cause you to say "screw it," which is when you'll proceed to binge eat anything your heart desires at that moment. And it's the binge eating that'll mess up your nutrition plan. Instead, a much better approach is to occasionally allow sweets or other treats in your diet from time to time.

Think about it, if it's in your diet plan to eat a small bowl of ice cream every three days, are you going to feel guilty when you eat that ice cream? No, you won't because it's part of the diet plan! On the flip side, if all junk food is forbidden under any circumstances, how are you going to feel if you eat a sweet treat? You'll feel horrible!

You'll feel like you cheated on your diet and that it's all over with. That, of course, isn't true, but in that moment, most people feel like complete failures. And this is one of the things I love most about the DASH diet. On the DASH diet eating plan, you're allowed to eat up to five servings of sweets per week.

This means that you won't have to completely give up your favorite sweet treats if you don't want to. The DASH diet is realistic about the fact that we're human. Seriously, who do you know of that could go the rest of their lives without eating another piece of junk food ever again? Probably no one! That's why the DASH diet is really not a diet as much as it's a lifestyle plan.

It's something that you'll easily be able to do for a very long time to come. This is great news when compared to other nutrition plans. Every day when you wake up, you think to yourself, "Dang another day of boring eating, I'm not sure how much longer I can handle this." And most people don't last long on boring diet plans that have them eating the same bland foods day in and day out.

With that being said, you'll of course want to limit certain food choices on the DASH diet. You can certainly include these things as part of your 5 servings of sweets per week but be cautious not to overdo it. The servings and calories can add up rather quickly if you do! This list isn't meant to scare you into not eating any of these foods, but rather to help you better understand why they need to be limited in order for you to be successful with the DASH diet plan.

Processed foods:

Processed foods are made with certain ingredients that will extend the shelf life of those foods. On one hand, this seems great. It allows the expiration date of a food item to be extended longer so we can take a longer time to eat the food if we wish.

However, we have to take a step back and consider the harmful effects these ingredients can have on our bodies over the long haul. Here are some reasons why you'll want to limit the consumption of processed foods:

Empty calories: processed foods in most cases contain a lot of empty calories. Imagine eating broccoli for example. This vegetable is rich in a lot of key vitamins and nutrients that your body needs. It doesn't contain a lot of calories, and the calories that it does contain are jam-packed with healthy nutrients.

On the flip side, consider a processed food item such as a candy bar. The candy bar doesn't contain very many beneficial vitamins and minerals for our bodies. It also contains a lot of calories from simple sugars. That's why the calories from something like a candy bar are considered to be empty. They're providing your body with nothing useful that it needs.

So, you'll likely be unable to get full and stay satisfied, meaning that you'll have to eat even more calories. This is why you must be cautious when eating processed foods. The calories won't do much to keep you full, and it can be very easy to overeat them.

High in trans-fat and processed oils: Remember that on the DASH diet we are seeking to eliminate or greatly limit the amount of trans fat that we're consuming. Most processed foods contain quite a bit of trans fat and processed oils that we'll want to avoid. These kinds of fats are high in Omega-6 fatty acids.

Omega-6 fatty acids by themselves are not bad, however they can become a problem when consumed in excess compared to Omega-3 fatty acids. Omega-6 fatty acids cause our bodies to become inflamed. Excess inflammation can cause damage to our joints, impede recovery, and cause heart disease among other things (14).

This is why it's important to have a balance of Omega-3 fatty acids, which act as an anti-inflammatory in the body. The Omega-3 fatty acids can help to counteract the inflammation from the Omega-6 fatty acids.

Low in fiber: processed foods contain a low amount of fiber. Other foods like fruits and vegetables contain high amounts of fiber. As I mentioned earlier, fiber is not only important for our digestive health, but it's also very important for keeping us full for longer periods of time.

This is the real danger of eating too many processed foods. They don't fill you up very well, so you have to eat more of them to get full. This likely means that you'll eat more calories than you should have.

Too many simple carbohydrates: Some people think that you should avoid carbs at all costs, and it's easy to believe considering how bad of a reputation carbs have been getting lately. However, all of this hate on carbs isn't justified. There are good carbs and bad carbs.

Not all carbs are evil and should be avoided like the plague. There are two different kinds of carbohydrates—simple and complex. Simple carbs are carbs that are quickly broken down and processed by the body. This is a bad thing because the rapid breakdown leads to a spike in your insulin levels.

Insulin spikes can lead to food cravings at random times, and your body doesn't burn fat while your insulin levels are high (15).

Conversely, there are complex carbohydrates. These are carbs such as brown rice and sweet potatoes. These kinds of carbs are slower digesting carbs that will not cause spikes in your blood sugar levels. Complex carbs are considered to be healthy carbs (in moderation of course). They also contain many beneficial vitamins and nutrients.

Sodas:

Sodas should be severely limited if not completely eliminated on the DASH diet. Limiting or eliminating soda intake is one of the first steps I have people take to start losing weight. The reason is similar to why you'd want to limit your intake of processed foods. Sodas contain an excessive amount of sugar, high fructose corn syrup, and empty calories.

Unlike certain processed foods, I consider soda and candy to be the ultimate forms of empty calories because they literally contain only sugar. They provide absolutely zero nutrition that's beneficial for your body. Soda and candy will do nothing to keep you full, and they'll give you random cravings—not good at all!

Excessive amounts of sugar have been linked to many negative health effects such as increased fat mass, increased amount of triglycerides in the blood, insulin resistance, and increase in low-density lipoproteins (the bad form of cholesterol) among other things (16). So needless to say, soda is something you'll definitely want to watch out for.

The thing is, sugar can be quite addicting (17), so how can you start to limit your soda intake if it's currently too high? I would avoid trying to quit cold turkey. Imagine if you've been drinking an average of two sodas per day for the last five years.

Is it really that likely you'll be able to walk away from it and never look back? Doubtful. Instead, you need to take a more steady approach. If, for example, you're drinking 16 ounces of soda per day, then start off by pouring out 4 ounces of the soda and diluting the remaining 12 ounces with 4 ounces of water.

After doing that for a week, take another step forward by pouring out 8 ounces of soda and diluting the remaining 8 ounces of soda with 8 ounces of water. From there, once that week has finished, you can do 4 ounces of soda with 12 ounces of water. And then move completely away from it.

Sure, it's tempting to want to go all out and eliminate soda completely in one fell swoop but know yourself and be wise. If you think you'd be more successful by being patient and gradually easing yourself off of soda, then do that.

Juices and other artificially sweetened beverages

Wait what? I thought things like orange juice were good for you? Yes, if you took oranges, squeezed them, and only drank the juice that came directly from the oranges that would be ok in moderation (although that'd be the equivalent of eating several oranges, so you'd want to factor that in to your daily servings of fruit).

However, most fruit juices and other artificially sweetened beverages aren't healthy options. The main reason is because they are loaded with a bunch of excessive sugar. Most juices don't contain purely the sugar found in the fruits.

Most of the time, there's added sugar in the juices. Yes, these juices do contain a lot of vitamins such as vitamin A and C, however this doesn't make them a healthy drink option. In fact, this deceives people into thinking that it's a healthy choice when the truth is that it's not.

If you want to get more vitamin A and C in your diet, then eat more fruits and vegetables. You don't have to go out of your way by drinking more fruit juices to get more vitamins. Yes, it's easier to consume these vitamins by drinking them, but it comes at a cost. And that cost is excessive amounts of sugar.

As mentioned earlier, too much sugar in the diet has been shown to lead to health problems such as metabolic syndrome, certain types of cancer, and diabetes. In addition to that, sugar has been shown to be highly addictive, so you must be careful with how much you consume. It's certainly best to avoid the unnecessary sugar and get your vitamins and nutrients from whole food sources such as fruits and vegetables.

If you really like tasty drinks, then consider consuming fruits and veggies in smoothie form without any added sugar. That way, you still get all the nutrients without the added sugars. Plus, when you make the smoothie yourself with fresh fruit and vegetables, you are getting more out of your food. When you purchase pre-made juices and fruits, studies have shown that many of these beverages start to lose their nutrients the longer they sit on the shelf. The sooner you can consume your fruits and veggies after preparing them, the better you'll be able to absorb the nutrients. That's one of the many

The Practical Dash Diet

great things about smoothies. If you can replace all sugary beverages with smoothies, you'll find tremendous improvements in your health. Also, smoothies can be a great way to kill a sweet tooth. Opt for a healthy smoothie instead of a milk shake. If you find a really fresh sweet pineapple, and make a smoothie with Greek yogurt and a minimal drizzle of honey, not only are you minimizing your calorie intake, but you're actually getting great nutrients from the fruit and yogurt. Instead of consuming 400 empty calories in a bowl of ice cream, you're consuming 200 nutritive and nourishing calories in the form of a healthy smoothie. And what's more, you'll feel satiated and satisfied and your cravings for sweets will have diminished or disappeared. The more you can train yourself to get used to this, the easier you'll find it.

White Bread

On the DASH diet, you're going to consuming whole grains, such as whole-wheat bread. Something you'll want to avoid is white bread. On the surface, it might appear as if bread is bread so what's the big deal with white bread? Why do we want to avoid eating it whenever possible?

For starters, white bread is a simple carbohydrate. As I mentioned earlier, simple carbs should be avoided in favor of complex carbs. Simple carbohydrates provide little nutritional value to your body, and they also cause rapid spikes in your blood sugar levels, which can lead to food cravings at random times throughout the day.

Not only that, but white bread ranks high on the glycemic index scale (GI scale for short). The GI scale measures how fast or slow different carbohydrates cause increases in blood glucose levels. The slower the carbohydrate increases blood glucose levels, the better it is, and thus the lower the score it'll receive on the glycemic index scale.

The scale ranges from 0-100, and basically what you need to know is that the closer a food item is to 0, the better it is for you. White bread has a GI score of 75 (18), which isn't good at all. It'll quickly raise blood sugar levels much faster than other carbohydrates will. That's why on the DASH diet, you'll be consuming whole grains, which rank much lower on the glycemic index scale. And you'll want to greatly limit or completely avoid carbs such as white bread.

French Fries

French fries are essentially the fried version of a potato. Now there's nothing wrong with a regular white potato or a sweet potato in moderation, however, when you take a potato and fry it, many things happen along the way that make the food item unhealthy. For instance, when the food is being cooked, it's being fried in unhealthy oils.

This is going to drastically increase the amount of fat content in the food. Not only that but when you order fries from a fast food restaurant, what are they going to add to the fries? That's right, they're going to add salt. This will unnecessarily increase the amount of sodium in the food.

And as you learned earlier, taking in too much sodium can cause hypertension, which is why you'll want to limit sodium intake on the DASH diet. Finally, fries are very easy to over consume. Think about how long it takes you to eat a potato or sweet potato. Now compare that to how long it takes you to wolf down a side of medium fries from a fast food restaurant.

And since these fries contain a lot of added fat, this means that they contain an excessive amount of calories as well. Plus, you won't be eating the fries plain as they are, of course you'll have to dip them in ketchup with contains high fructose corn syrup and more sugar than you'd think. Fries are definitely something you can overeat rather quickly, so be very cautious of this food on the DASH diet.

Cookies, cakes, and other pastries

These sweet treats are another simple carbohydrate that you'll want to watch out for. Their nutritional content is made up primarily of refined sugars and other processed ingredients. These foods usually contain shortening, which is a type of solid fat that's high in saturated fat. This is one of the bad types of fat that you'll want to limit whenever possible. Yes, these foods are tasty, but be wary not to over consume them as part of your 5 servings per week following the nutritional plan

The Practical Dash Diet

Make Gradual Changes

Gradually make healthier choices to your dieting plan. You're not going to change your entire way of life in a single day, so plan for small changes that gradually move you in the right direction. The reason that so many people fail is that they try to make changes that are unrealistic. Rather than setting yourself up for failure, start small.

- Make one or two small changes every day.
- Replace an unhealthy choice with fresh veggies for lunch.
- Add a serving of fruit to your meal, or better yet, replace a snack with fruit.
- Swap to whole grain bread.
- Switch to whole grain, no added sugar cereal.
- Rather than filling your plate with food, opt for a smaller portion.
- Experiment with healthy recipes by adding a new one every week. Write down your favorites, and slowly replace less healthy meal plans with those healthy ones.
- If you love ice cream, choose low-fat frozen yogurt instead.
- Replace sugary drinks with club soda or water or fresh fruit and veggie smoothies. This one is a huge step!
- When you get a sweet tooth, opt for fruit over processed snacks. You can eat canned fruit as long as it's not packed in syrup. Look at the label.

The DASH diet is focused on whole grains, vegetables, and fruit, so you need to gradually incorporate those into your lifestyle. Additionally, you will also need to start reducing your food portions. Instead of just piling food onto your plate, start measuring out one serving of each food.

Make sure that you slowly incorporate fiber into your diet. Adding too much fiber too quickly will make you feel bloated and can lead to diarrhea. These symptoms are not unhealthy. It's your body detoxifying itself, but it could really test your patience. We want this to be easy.

If you are lactose intolerant, then you can opt for lactose-free products rather than dairy. If you're allergic to nuts, then choose seeds or legumes instead. This is not some super strict plan like so many others before it. The idea is to make a lifestyle change. Those take more time and commitment but become much easier the longer you do them. Fad diets get more difficult as you continue, which is why they fail more often than not.

Limit Meat Consumption

If you are an avid consumer of meat, then you should start cutting back on it. Try only eating two servings of meat per day. This actually has two major advantages. One is that it's a healthy choice. Second is that meatless meals are often much more budget-friendly. Try going meatless once or twice a week–basing your diet around plant-based proteins like beans, lentils, vegetables, and whole grains.

Plant-based meals are loaded with vitamins and important nutrients. Did you know that vegetarians consume fewer calories on average than meat eaters? Now, I'm not saying that you need to start living a vegetarian or vegan lifestyle, only that you make a small change to the way you look at food. You do not need more than two servings of meat per day, especially when there are so many healthy choices out there.

How much protein is enough? You only need 50 grams of protein per day at the most, so cutting back on meat is not going to hurt you.

Additionally, you can replace fatty meats (red meat) with leaner meats like fish and poultry. Again, don't do this all at once. Start by reducing your meat servings per day by one serving until you work your way down to two per day. Then after a few weeks, you can start to add in meatless days until you are at two.

Substitute Healthy Desserts

You should immediately replace all of your sugary, processed dessert choices with dried, fresh, or canned fruits. Fruit is sweet but is loaded with other healthy nutrients. For example, most processed desserts do not have Vitamin A or Vitamin C, both of which are essential vitamins for the body.

Fruit also provides nutrients like fiber and folic acid. So next time you get a sweet tooth, bypass those baked goods, and try eating a piece of fruit. In fact, berries will give you the added bonus of an energy boost. It's a neat trick that nutritionists use to help their clients with that afternoon energy crash.

Nutrients provided by fruit are so important to your body that they simply cannot be ignored. The easiest way to incorporate them into your daily life is to use them as a dessert treat. Here are some of the many benefits of fruit:

➤ Diets rich in fruit can reduce the risk for stroke, cardiovascular disease, and Type-2 diabetes.

➤ Fruit-rich diets can reduce the risk of certain cancer.

➤ Fruits promote phytochemicals, which will promote and maintain your overall health.

You only have to consume one to two cups of fruit each day to reap in the benefits, so making this small change will probably get your health on the right track.

Reduce Oils

This one is actually quite easy. Reduce the oils that you use when cooking by half. Almost everyone overuses oils for cooking, so this reduction is quite easy. It will improve the quality of your food. Oil is bad for two important reasons:

1: Oil is Pure Fat

Even olive oil is pure fat, so you should use as little as possible. It doesn't offer any real nutritional value, even though it's a good alternative. Marketers love to try to convince you otherwise, but you are basically consuming concentrated calories. My point is that we all use way too much oil because it's easy to do. That's why it's so important to measure it.

2: Oil Lacks Nutrients

Again, it's just a concentrated mixture of calories. It has no vitamins or minerals that help you at all. All healthy elements are left out when it's processed. However, you still need to use it in order to cook efficiently. That's why we use olive oil in our recipes. The key is to use as little as possible. With that said, you can also use raw and cold-pressed oils since a lot of the nutrients are preserved. Again, these are simple changes that require minimal effort.

Increase Your Dairy Intake

Today's society pushes sugary beverages at us like they are the best thing in the world! But they are actually the opposite. Marketing focuses on the emotions attached to these sugary drinks to blind us from the fact that they are poison. You are going to have to get rid of these drinks if you plan on living a healthy life. There is no wiggle-room here.

So, let's make this easier on you by replacing all sodas and other sugar-filled drinks with fat-free milk. Try getting at least three servings in every day. I read so many Internet "experts" write about swearing off dairy products, but that's not a good choice. The only dairy products I recommend you stay away from are whole fat-filled ones.

➢ Dairy contains calcium, which helps promote bone mass and healthy teeth. Three servings of milk daily will provide you with enough calcium.

➢ Certain dairy products, like yogurt provide potassium.

➢ Vitamin D is another nutrient with amazing benefit to the body as it also helps with bone development. Milk is a great source of Vitamin D.

➢ Skim milk produces endorphins in the brain much the same way as soda, but it also provides important nutrients. You might still get the calories, but at least those calories are not wasted.

➢ Dairy products have been linked to a reduction in the risk of cardiovascular disease.

➢ Certain dairy products have high levels of saturated fat, which will actually have a negative impact on your health. That's why this book tells you to choose from the low-fat/fat-free choices.

The Power of the Dash Diet

I. The Positive Impact of Dash Diet

The Dash Diet is known for being a FAMILY-oriented Diet. It can be adopted by individuals of all ages right from kids to adults to the older members, this nutrition plan takes care of the overall health of the family. Of course always consult your doctor before starting any new diet plan and of course if Children are involved you'll want to clear it with their Pediatrician.

1.) A Wholesome Diet – Dash Diet

Dash Diet promotes consuming all three macronutrients – *carbs, proteins and fats.* The idea behind the diet is to take care of your primary meals – *breakfast, lunch and dinner* along with your *snacking needs* throughout the day. In a diet like this you tend to eat all kinds of healthy foods which in turn reduces your chance/desire of eating junk or unhealthy food items.

2.) Take Control of Your Blood Pressure

Life these days is stressful and it can get really difficult to stick to a meal plan, let alone a nutrition plan. The consumption of whole grains, fruits and vegetables help in reducing hunger especially when taken in small quantities throughout the day. Potassium, calcium and magnesium filled foods work as crucial elements to stabilize the levels of blood pressure.

Now, many people are unclear about the quantities of sodium that our body requires. So, you may ask me, isn't sodium as important as the other elements of nutrition?

Well, yes, it is! Sodium is an essential element for our body and our sodium intake is a concern more than a question. The Dash Diet is designed in a way that it gives you the right amount of sodium which eases critical body functions and does not allow additional fluids to increase. High amounts of sodium can cause extra fluids to build which in turn raises your blood pressure.

The NIH has revealed that the Dash Diet can bring down an individual's blood pressure in JUST 14 days – **Amazing Fact**

3.) The NEW Added Benefit of the Dash Diet –Cholesterol Management

For some reason, the Dash Diet is known to be one of the MOST RESEARCHED topics of its kind. Researchers found out that this diet does not just help you lower your BP but also supports you in managing your cholesterol levels. How, you may ask? *Fibers* play a significant role in managing one's cholesterol levels. The foods consumed as per Dash nutrition plans includes whole wheat items such as brown rice, oats, barley, millet and similar others which are a great source of fiber.

Recently, there was an interesting twist in a Dash study which stated that the consumption of high-fat dairy products in the diet could actually lower bad cholesterol levels in individuals who were affected. Hey! Hang on there, before you call me nuts for contradicting myself let me tell you something: in addition to the new findings it was also noticed that two individuals who followed the Dash diet with two different patterns of consuming high-fat and low-fat dairy products got the same results of reduced blood pressure. Now, that's what I call the magic of DASH!!

Health Tip: *The proper fiber portion for men can range from 30 to 38 grams per day whereas for women it could be between 20 to 25 grams per day.*

4.) The Weight Management Plan

The Dash Diet has emerged as a weight loss plan over the period of years and is said to have a great impact on individuals who are struggling with weight issues such as obesity. There is no denial that apart from its prime motive of minimizing heart problems by reducing your blood pressure the Dash Diet has measurable effects on one's weight. The consumption of fruits and vegetables at regular intervals keeps you full and in turn helps you keep a check on your calorie intake. However, if you are looking for a quick overnight weight loss solution, you may be out of luck. This is a slow and steady process that will contribute to overall better health as well as significant weight loss.

II. The Complexities of the Dash Diet

Complexities? Did you just say complexities Cage? Yes, I did! Unfortunately, every diet has its own drawbacks and the Dash Diet is no different. While this diet gets two thumbs up from the best health organizations of the world there are two complexities I want to bring to your notice,

1.) Taste Issues – Where's the SALT?

For those families and individuals who have always preferred less SALT in their food, they will not face a problem at all. But for the ones who are used to adding SALT to their cooked meals this diet can put you through an irritable moment. Initially you may find it difficult to cope with the taste but gradually you will manage to get your head around it. Believe me, a little persistence here can give you immense benefits. Plus you will find ways to be creative and season your food without loading it up with salt. There are many ways to enhance the flavor of your food, salt just happens to be the most popular. Using many herbs and spices as well as a lot of citrus will make your food taste amazing without maxing out the sodium content.

2.) Calorie Check – The Ups and Downs

Gruesome! This one's certainly horrifying and yes, I have been through it. The older me literally carried a checklist and meter just to ensure I didn't consume a bit more than what was supposed to be eaten. Oh well, that is history! But, you know the formulation of DASH Diet is quite precise and all you need is a proper nutrition form based on your lifestyle. I'd recommend not going overboard with calorie checking because it can get in the way of what you're actually trying to do here.

DASH Diet FAQ

Is the DASH diet only for hypertension?

No. although it was designed for people with hypertension, the diet has been adopted by several other groups for its benefits in ameliorating their health conditions. This includes people who are trying to lose weight, build lean muscle, etc. Along with a substantial reduction in weight, DASH dieters also see their hypertension reduced, which helps them lead happy lives free from stress and illness.

Does it follow a phase system?

Yes. It follows a two-phase system where the first phase completely eliminates foods that are starchy and laden with carbohydrates and the second phase slowly reintroduces them. This system helps the person's body cope with the diet so they can continue with it for a long time. The two phases have a difference of 2 weeks between them, and that is the time when dieters are said to experience the greatest amount of weight loss.

Is it good for losing weight?

Yes. This diet is said to be quite effective in helping people lose weight. It is said to be on par with some of the other diets that are prescribed specifically for weight loss, and if followed the right way, it can have the same results on people's bodies. The diet is quite effective not just in helping a person lose weight but also in keeping that weight from coming back. The diet can be seen as your one-stop, ultra-effective means to cut down on excess weight and maintain a healthy body.

Is the DASH diet for all ages?

The diet can be followed by people above the age of 18. Children below that age might need foods rich in carbs and salt for proper growth. Anybody else looking to reduce their high blood pressure and hypertension and cut down on their weight can take up the diet. There is no upper age limit for the diet. However, older people need to check with their doctors first to know if it will be safe for them to take up the diet.

Is it ideal for busy professionals?

Yes. The diet will work well for busy professionals as they will have the opportunity to prepare the meals in advance. Preparing their meals in advance on weekends will help them save time and effort on busy weekdays. The recipes in this book are great for busy professionals who seek to use the DASH diet to lessen their hypertension and reduce their weight.

Are the results fast?

The results will depend on how seriously you take the diet – whether you are strictly following the rules of the diet and are incorporating only the allowed food items. The results can usually be seen within the first month of the diet, but it will vary from person to person. It can be fast for some and might take some more time for others. If you are taking up the diet with another person, then it is best that you not compare your results with theirs and focus only on your diet.

Are the results noticeable?

Yes. The results are quite easy to see, and you will feel that your blood pressure has dropped and your metabolism is now much better. You will feel a physical change and feel lighter after taking up the diet. The diet will also help you maintain a slim figure and give you a chance to build lean, strong muscles. You will see a reduction in your waistline, and this will help bring down your blood pressure. You will feel much more energetic and capable of doing physical tasks without exerting too much pressure on your heart.

Is it suitable for vegetarians?

Although the diet calls for the consumption of quite a bit of meat, it is also suited for vegetarians. There are many vegetarian super foods which will help offset the lack of meat in the diet, and vegetarians will be able to make the switch quite comfortably.

Is it sustainable?

Yes. The diet can be continued for life; there will be no negative impact on the body. You can choose to go off the diet for a couple of months and take it up again later. You need not stop it just because you have attained your ideal body weight; you can continue to follow it to maintain your body weight. You might try taking it up for a month, and if the results are satisfactory, continuing with it for the rest of your life.

DASH Tips for Busy People

Trying to cram all your activities into a 24-hour day leaves very little time for food preparation. A busy lifestyle leads people to rely on fast food for their meals. Unfortunately, the most convenient solution for busy people can also be the unhealthiest option. Junk food has too much sodium, sugar and fat, and consuming it regularly can lead to many health issues like obesity and diabetes. The best approach to staying healthy even during hectic days is to plan ahead and acquire as much nutritional knowledge as possible.

Stock up on nutritional snacks

Nuts and granola bars are far better options than chips and cookies. Carry healthy snacks to work and avoid relying on the vending machine for food. It's easy to be tempted to eat delicious but unhealthy food right after a busy work day. Having a stash of healthy snacks at home will lessen the urge to stop by the fast food chain. You can use a Sunday to make a large batch of these healthy snacks. Just store them in containers and decide which one you'll consume each day. Remember that you can make your own granola bars as well with a little patience. Homemade is always a better choice than store-bought, as you will be aware of the good quality ingredients that have gone into making the item. The same cannot be said about factory-made foods. So, no matter what the food item is, consider making it yourself. Only if that's too tedious should you consider buying it from the store.

Stick to your list

People benefit from mastering their grocery shopping. Try to list all the supplies needed for an entire week so that you'll spend less time on shopping. Try to stick to the list and avoid wandering off to the processed food section of the grocery store to avoid impulsive buying. You can also enlist the help of a friend or your partner when you go shopping. Not only will it take you less time to finish, but you'll also have help in staying away from the processed foods. Once you have a list that works for you, use the same one every week and simply add or subtract any relevant ingredients based on your planned menu for that week. You can also opt to shop online; that might make it easier to stay away from unnecessary foods than if you're physically present in a store. This will also save you the to and fro journey, and you can even shop from your office.

Befriend your refrigerator

Cook meals that can be refrigerated. This way, you only have to cook once and the dish can last for at least a few days. Set aside a few hours on Sunday nights to prepare meals for the week. Cook, divide into portions, and refrigerate. This is the same thing as cutting your vegetables in bulk and placing them under cling film. Adding a little vinegar will help preserve your dishes longer, and you need not rely on salt to help your meals stay fresh. You must, however, remember to heat the food thoroughly before consuming it, as sitting in the fridge might cause germ growth. One good idea is to prepare and store the main courses and make a fresh salad to go with them each night. That way, you will not have everything coming out of your fridge – it will be a combination of reheated and fresh.

Be creative in transforming leftovers

Protein foods like chicken and pork can be reinvented in a number of ways. Although salads are the go-to dishes for leftovers, meat can be used in tortillas or sliced into small bits and added to low-sodium, low-fat mayonnaise for a sandwich. There are many different possibilities for leftovers; it is up to you to creatively transform one food into another to avoid getting bored eating the same dish over and over again. However, your leftovers will remain fresh only so long, and it is best to use today's leftovers only for the next couple of days.

Hydrate

Busy people tend to forget to drink enough liquid, and oftentimes if they do drink, they choose soda or an energy drink. These contain too much sugar and can contribute to developing hypertension or diabetes. Also, watch out for calories inside commercially prepared drinks such as fruit juices, sweet or carbonated tea, and canned coffee. They also contain too much sugar and have a lot of empty calories which can sabotage any diet plan. If your workplace does not have a water cooler for employees, bring a water bottle to work filled with water or plain tea. You can also choose fruit infused water, which serves the dual purpose of providing your body with the goodness of fresh fruits and water. All you have to do is place the fresh fruit (kiwi, strawberry, orange etc.) along with a few fresh herbs (mint, basil, rosemary etc.) in a container and pour in enough water to cover them. Use a muddler or a spatula to bash the fruit and herbs so they release their flavors and pour the infused water into a bottle after straining it. This water can be freshened up by adding a few ice cubes and some lemon water and drinking it regularly will help flush out all the toxins from your body.

Fitness

When it comes to controlling your blood pressure, it is important to exercise regularly. This helps in reducing the amount of pressure that is exerted on the heart. Remember that your heart needs exercise and you must engage in cardio to give it a thorough burn. Many people refrain from undertaking cardio exercise as they think it will tire them out completely. But the main aim of cardio is to exhaust you and help you achieve a burn. Apart from cardio, you must also do other forms of exercise, including lifting weights, core training, sides, back muscle stimulation, etc. After you do these, your body will be able to pump blood through your heart more easily.

Apart from reducing your total body weight, it is also important to reduce your waistline. Some people neglect their waistline and start concentrating on their arms and back. But these don't have much of a bearing on your heart; it's important to concentrate on your stomach area. Pushups, pull-ups, planks and crunches will do your waist a lot of good.

How to find time for fitness

Finding time for fitness routines is always a choice. It can be quite challenging to fit an exercise regimen in between work and household errands, but it is not impossible. Remember that physical fitness combined with healthy diet is the key to balanced physical and emotional health and try to exercise as often as you can to get the most out of your regimen. This does not always have to mean hitting the gym. There are many ways in which you can get a thorough burn just by making use of the workout opportunities that you are presented with in your day-to-day life.

Make workouts fit into your current lifestyle

Parents: Try to spend quality time with your kids outdoors. Take a bike ride around the park or schedule hiking trips. Such activities keep the body fit and the family bonded. You can decide on a day in advance and ask all your family members to be ready for it. Parents can also take up a sport such as playing basketball with their children, teaching them to swim, etc.

Students: Visit the school gym during breaks. Take advantage of school privileges instead of spending money on gym memberships outside. Taking up sports is also a great idea. Take up basketball or join the athletics team to shed weight and maintain a lean body.

Young professionals: Work out before breakfast, which will give you some quiet time to think and reflect before you're submerged again into a busy work life. You can get up a little early and take a brisk walk. You can then start jogging and eventually take up running. If you do not have an open area near you, you can do some aerobics in your house or room.

You can also take up a fun activity such as dancing or swimming; both will help you shed excess weight in no time. Belly dancing is great for women, and men can take up salsa. You can get your partner to join in – join a foxtrot or tango class together.

Listen to your body

Your body will often give clues about what exercise it needs. People with desk jobs will find rigorous activities like running and kickboxing a refreshing chance to release pent-up energy. People who have physically demanding jobs can benefit from yoga and long walks to help calm their minds. Take up the best type of exercise for yourself depending on your line of business. But if you keep doing the same old thing over and over again, your muscles will start to tire and you might end up with muscle loss. So, try and switch up the exercises that you undertake and introduce as much variety as possible.

Make fitness a must

Make no room for excuses and prioritize your fitness regimen. The main area that you need to focus on is your waistline, as a large one will keep your blood pressure high. Make a commitment to keep your body fit and healthy as long as possible. Placing Post-it® Notes to remind yourself of fitness goals will help you stay on track. You can also make use of alarms and reminders to help you exercise every day. Some people prefer to time their exercise regime with something that they always do so it's easier to remember. Once you start, maintain a consistent record so that you will remain motivated to carry on with your exercise routine. From time to time you can reward yourself with something nice for the good work that you do.

Other lifestyle choices

Remember that the DASH diet will not work unless you supplement it with proper exercise and refrain from bad lifestyle choices. Some things to consider:

When on the diet, you must refrain from consuming junk foods and processed foods as both are laden with salts and unnecessary carbs. They also contain chemicals that can be bad for your body.

The next thing is to quit indulging in bad habits such as drinking and smoking. Drinking excess alcohol can cause your heart to weaken. Binge drinking can cause your blood pressure to surge, which can have dangerous consequences. Smoking will also block your arteries, and this can be bad for your heart. Remember that secondary smoke is as bad as primary. If someone in your house or office smokes, ask them to stop or move away.

Excess intake of caffeine can cause your blood pressure to surge. High blood pressure can cause your heart to suffer, so it is important to either quit drinking caffeinated drinks or limit it to just a cup a day.

You must also reduce your stress to a bare minimum in order to fight high blood pressure. You can take up meditation and indulge in yoga to reduce everyday tensions. You can also take up a hobby such as dancing or singing to limit your stress.

Positive actions

If you are following the diet to help with your high blood pressure, then you can monitor your blood pressure at home from time to time. You can buy yourself a machine and check if the diet is working for you. If there is a positive outcome just continue with your diet, but if there is no visible change you should modify your diet a little.

You can join a support group to help you reduce your stress. You will be in the company of others who are affected by the same issues you are, and you will find it easier to cope with your condition. You can look online for a class or ask acquaintances if they know of any. If there is no such group in your locality then you can start one yourself. You can invite others who suffer from the same condition and conduct regular meetings.

Why the DASH diet is sustainable

The DASH diet is sustainable because it does not impose too many restrictions on the dieter. Although it is known as a "diet", it does not limit intake to salads and juices. There is a lot of variety that can be incorporated in terms of flavors and ingredients, and there will be no danger of monotony setting in.

Another advantage of the diet is that it does not impose portion restrictions. There is no restriction on how much food can be consumed at one time and since the meals that are prepared are healthy, the body can digest as much food as it is provided with.

The low sodium content in the diet means that dieters don't feel thirsty all the time. This helps them consume more healthy and nutritious food instead of filling up on water. Less salt also means the kidneys and liver will remain healthy and there will be no excessive pressure on the heart.

The diet will show quick results in terms of weight loss as the excess fiber content will increase the body's metabolism. This will cause the person's digestive tract to function optimally and the body will start burning fat. From the liquids to the sides, almost everything in the diet is high in fiber. That makes it great for increasing your metabolic rate.

One of the biggest advantages of this diet is that it supplies the body with just the right amount of energy for it to conduct day-to-day activities. No excess energy is available for the body to store as fat, and this helps DASH dieters remain slim.

The high protein content in the diet helps build strong muscles. With strong muscles, it is possible to burn away fat with ease and there is no room for fat storage. So, this diet is great for those trying to build a muscular body.

The Practical Dash Diet

Dash Kitchen:

Just as you need to select the ingredients you know you will use, select kitchen equipment you are comfortable with. The recipes in this book require a minimum amount of equipment, while still taking advantage of labor-saving devices. Make your kitchen a friendly, welcoming, organized place. Your time in the kitchen should be pleasant and it should be easy for you to prep and prepare meals. The following two lists include essential equipment and nice-to-have equipment.

Essential Equipment

This list of essential equipment includes items needed for daily cooking, aimed at the beginner cook:

Nonstick skillet or frying pan with lid. A good nonstick skillet is indispensable, making it easy to brown, fry, and sauté. Choose a size that works for you according to the number of people in your household.

A small and a large pot, with lids. A small and a large saucepan will be used in this book to prepare sauces, soups, and stews. Choosing ones with a nonstick coating will make clean up easy and won't require a lot of oil when using. Nontoxic eco-friendly options include glass, ceramic, stainless steel, and green nonstick cookware.

Baking dishes. Glass or metal baking dishes are used for roasting meats and preparing casserole-type dishes. They are even useful for serving straight from the oven to the table and can be used to store leftovers.

Rimmed 9-by-13-inch baking sheet. A baking sheet with a 1-inch rim is designed to catch juices from roasting vegetables, meats, fish, and poultry. Choose from metal or silicone.

Knives. The two most important knives for efficient prep in the kitchen are a good-quality chef's knife for larger items, like meats, and a paring knife for fruits, vegetables, and herbs.

Cutting boards. A wooden cutting board will be easy on kitchen knives, keeping them sharp for longer. Dedicated cutting boards are ideal—one for fresh vegetables and fruits, one for meats—but this isn't always practical on a tight budget. If you are using one cutting board, be sure to avoid cross-contamination by sanitizing your board after working with raw meats and seafood.

Assorted mixing bowls. Look for durable nesting bowls that can handle large and small volumes. Look for bowls with lids, which can be used for storing leftovers.

Blender. A basic blender is needed to make smoothies and can also take the place of a food processor for puréeing soups and beans. Try to purchase one with at least 450 watts of power so you have the flexibility you need to effortlessly process a variety of ingredients.

The Practical Dash Diet

Nice-to-Have Equipment

Food processor. A food processor is nice to have for chopping, slicing, grating, dicing, and puréeing a variety of ingredients including nuts, beans, soups, vegetables, and grains. Food processors are similar to blenders but they have interchangeable blades and discs rather than a fixed blade.

Spiralizer. A spiralizer turns fresh veggies into faux noodles. Most models are about the size of a large toaster and function like a giant pencil sharpener. Spiralizing veggies and using them in place of pasta is a great way to boost your intake of vegetables while cutting back on calories.

Slow cooker. A slow cooker has many advantages and is a great way to save time while preparing a nutritious meal. Slow cookers can be used for breakfast casseroles, steel-cut oats, soups, stews, roasts, and grains.

The Practical Dash Diet

Dash Shopping

Tips for Using DASH When Shopping and Cooking
We have already recommended that you become a perimeter shopper to the greatest extent possible because that helps you to avoid buying those jars of sauce, packaged meals, and other foods that are literally saturated with sodium.

What can you purchase on the perimeter? Use this recommended DASH shopping list to help you stock your shelves and make the DASH lifestyle easier to follow. There are some canned and pre-made foods in the list, but note that all are marked as "low sodium", "fat free", etc.

DASH Shopping List

Vegetables:
- Artichokes
- Asparagus
- Avocados
- Beets
- Bell peppers
- Broccoli
- Brussels sprouts
- Cabbage
- Carrots
- Cauliflower
- Celery
- Corn
- Cucumbers
- Eggplant
- Green beans
- Leafy greens
- Leeks
- Mushrooms
- Onions
- Peas
- Potatoes
- Radishes
- Root vegetables
- Spinach
- Squash
- Tomatoes

Fruits
- Apples
- Apricots
- Bananas
- Berries
- Cherries
- Oranges
- Dates
- Figs
- Grapefruit
- Grapes
- Kiwi
- Lemons
- Limes
- Mango
- Melons
- Peaches
- Papaya
- Pears
- Pineapple
- Plums
- Prunes

Protein Sources
- Beef
- Chicken (skinless)
- Eggs
- Pork tenderloin
- Salmon
- Shrimp
- Tempeh
- Tofu
- Turkey (skinless)

Grains
- Barley
- Bran Cereal
- Brown rice
- Bulgur
- Couscous (whole wheat)
- Kasha (buckwheat)
- Low fat granola
- Muesli
- Pasta (Whole Wheat or Brown Rice)
- Quinoa, Millet, Amaranth
- Spelt, Triticale, Kamut
- Steel Cut Oats
- Whole Grain Cereal
- Wild rice

Dairy
- Buttermilk (low fat)
- Cheese
- Cottage cheese (low fat)
- Kefir
- Margarine
- Milk (low fat)
- Sour cream (low fat)
- Yogurt (low fat)

Nuts and Seeds
- Almonds
- Cashews
- Hazelnuts
- Nut butter
- Peanuts
- Pecans
- Seeds
- Soy nuts
- Walnut

Accepted Canned Goods
- Applesauce (unsweeten)
- Beans and lentils
- Broth (low sodium)
- Chiles (diced)

- Chili sauce or hot sauce (low sodium)
- Fresh salsa or Pico de gallo (low sodium)
- Fruit-only or low-sugar spreads
- Hummus (low sodium)
- Marinara sauce (low sodium)
- Mayonnaise (low-fat)
- Mustard (low sodium)
- Oil: canola, olive, sesame
- Pesto (low sodium)
- Salad dressing (low fat)
- Salmon or tuna (in water)
- Soup (low sodium)
- Soy sauce (low sodium)
- Sun-dried tomatoes
- Tomato paste (low sodium)

- Tomato sauce (low sodium)
- Tomatoes (low sodium)
- Vinegar

Helpful Extras:

- Herbs (dried and fresh)
- Spices of all kinds (skip any blends that use sodium or MSG)
- Popcorn to be used in an air popper
- Dried fruits
- Herbal tea
- Sodium-free vegetable juices
- No sugar fruit juices (be sure they are 100% fruit)
- Sparkling water (a reasonable alternative to soda)

The Practical Dash Diet

Eating Out on the Dash Diet:

Socializing over meals is very common across cultures. Now-a-days, this socializing occurs at a table in a restaurant. Whether you can eat out or not during the regime strictly depends upon the type of the restaurant and the food that you order. If you make intelligent choices from the menu and give some handy instructions to the waiter, then yes, you can eat out. However, if you are not sure, then it is not worth the risk.

Dash Diet for Weight Loss

Even though this dieting plan was created for the sole purpose of lowering blood pressure and getting a handle on cholesterol, we're going to adapt it in a way that also makes it a powerful weight-loss tool. This dieting plan already puts an emphasis on eating food that is low in cholesterol and saturated fat. The fact that it will have you eating more whole foods will lead to a certain amount of weight-loss automatically.

What we're going to do is take the DASH diet and make a few minor tweaks to make it more efficient for losing weight.

Keep a Food Journal

Having a food journal gives you an easy way to go back to review your food consumption periodically. Write down every meal you eat and place a timestamp on it. This includes snacks and drinks—everything you put into your body should be documented. Take it a step further and document your activity while eating. For example, "I had popcorn while watching a movie."

It's easy to lose track of your food consumption, so documenting it gives you an easy way to go back and review it on a weekly basis. You can see where you stand in terms of your eating habits, so you can start fixing the bad ones.

Calculate Your Calorie Goal

If you are planning to lose weight, then you will have to lower your calorie intake, so that it's less than what you burn on a daily basis. But you must do it gradually so that it doesn't throw your metabolism out of whack.

Start out by determining exactly what activities you perform on a daily basis.

When you determine how many calories you are burning per day, then you need to develop a plan. Here's an example:

You are burning 1,200 calories per day, so you will set up a list of goals as follows:

Week 1: 2,000 calories per day.

Week 2: 1,600 calories per day.

The primary goal of the diet is not actually for weight loss, but with the demand for an effective diet plan that can also solve different health problems, a new DASH Diet research has been conducted to further optimize the present diet plan. Carbs that are not nutritionally balanced were eliminated and more protein-rich food and heart healthy fats were added in the diet, resulting in an effective weight loss diet plan. There are two phases

The Practical Dash Diet

in the diet. Phase One is for the first 14 days of the diet, while Phase Two comes in after 2 weeks in the diet.

Phase 1: Shed Weight Two Weeks

During these 14 days you will learn how to satisfy your hunger with DASH Diet approved foods and as a result, you will feel fuller for a longer time. While whole grains, starchy veggies and fruits are included in the DASH Diet, it's advised that you eliminate these food groups first in the first two weeks of the diet; doing this will help regulate your blood sugar levels and will also curb your cravings for food. Milk is should also be avoided, but you can however, get at least moderated servings of non-fat yogurt. (Don't worry, you'll be able to re-introduce these foods back into your diet in moderate quantities later).

Amp up your consumption of green veggies such as spinach or other vegetables like broccoli, or cabbage, as well as other vegetables such as cucumbers, peppers and tomatoes.

You can also enjoy up to six ounces of lean meats, fish and poultry a day. Aim for four to five servings of beans or lentils a week.

Be wise in choosing your sources of fat. The best way to do this is by eating fish rich in healthy fats such as salmon and mackerel, or by using oils such as olive oil, and almond oil. Absolutely avoid foods that contain saturated and trans fats such as whole-fat dairy, fried foods, vegetable shortening, and store-bought pastries.

Phase 2: Kick It Up a Notch!

After the first 14 days, you will continue eating the foods from Phase 1 but you may start eating some other healthy foods that will help you continue your weight loss. You any choose the following food groups:

Whole Grains: Choose from breads and pasta, cereals, or any items made with whole grain. And totally eliminate foods made from refined grains such as white bread and pasta because these foods cause your blood sugar levels to spike. You can have six to eight servings of whole grains a day.

Fruit: Either fresh or frozen, you should aim to consume four to five servings of fruits daily.

Low-Fat Milk or Yogurt: These are great sources of calcium and Vitamin D. for your body in order to give you strong muscles and bones and also keep your metabolism working.

Sugar-Sugar and other sweets are now allowed in this phase as long as you limit it to not more than five servings a day.

Alcohol- alcohol in the form of wine is allowed in phase two as long as you limit it to a small glass occasionally.

If you really want to live and healthy for the rest of your life, I suggest the you follow the meal plan in phase two and you'll see that you'll be reaping the benefits of DASH Diet in no time.

The Practical Dash Diet

Make the Transition Slowly

When you make too many changes all at once, you will destabilize your body. This makes you crave your old diet and leads to relapses. It's extremely difficult to fight off your body's survival instincts, and that's exactly what your body does when it's in shock. It believes that survival is at risk, so it creates irresistible urges.

That's why it's important to make the transition slowly. Pace yourself by adapting to your new dietary plan so that your body doesn't even notice. You will eventually experience a full change and wonder how you ever led an unhealthy lifestyle.

Reduce Your Consumption of Fat and Sugar Even Further

Even though the DASH diet is going to have you reducing trans and saturated fat intake, in order to lose weight, you will need to avoid/reduce all types of fat in the beginning. Once you have reached your weight goal, then you can gradually work your way back up to the normal fats.

Stick to poultry and fish as your primary sources of meat. You should probably limit meat to once every day. Replace it with vegetables that are high in protein.

You will also need to reduce the sugars that you consume, including fruits in the beginning, if you want to lose weight. You should limit fruit consumption to one serving per day. Take a multi-vitamin to make up for the loss of nutrients. Once you have reached your weight loss goal, you can start to enjoy fruits as normal again.

Limit Sodium to 1,500 mg per Day

Remember when I said there were two types of DASH diet plans? You are going to want to opt for the one with less sodium intake. This is an area where so many people mess up when losing weight. They do everything right, except keeping their sodium intake down. Then they don't lose weight because the sodium causes their body to retain more water.

The main way to lower your sodium is by avoiding meats that are high in sodium. You will need to pay close attention to labels.

Eat More Vegetables and Whole Grains

Weight loss requires a few additional steps, one of which is to eat even more vegetables. Since you will need to reduce meat and sugar consumption in the initial stages, you will have to replace them with vegetables and whole grains. When I say whole grains, I mean everything–rice and noodles included.

Again, when using canned vegetables be sure that you read the label because some of those items are loaded with sodium and added sugar. Just keep in mind that you need to make these changes gradually to avoid shocking your system.

The Practical Dash Diet

Fat-Free is Not Always Healthy

Fat-free does not always mean that a product is healthy. For example, some fat-free salad dressings contain even more calories than their fat-filled counterparts! That's why it's so important to read labels.

Most people will just blindly trust that the words "fat-free" mean healthier. That is simply not always the case.

Distribute Your Calories Throughout the Day

Eating smaller portions of food throughout the entire day will help your body burn calories more efficiently because of the metabolic boost that accompanies it. If you are eating a super large dinner, then spread that meal throughout the entire day. Usually, people who eat huge dinners skip lunch, which is a huge mistake.

Eating smaller portions is the absolute best habit you can develop for losing weight. Just this one change makes a huge difference. You should follow a specific meal pattern. The more consistent you are, the more efficient your body will function.

➢ Breakfast

➢ Morning snack

➢ Lunch

➢ Afternoon snack

➢ Dinner

➢ After-dinner snack (at least two hours before bed)

One of the final weight-loss tips for adding to the DASH diet is to exercise regularly, so the next chapter is dedicated to exercise.

Exercise Plan

Now we're going to move onto a topic that drives so many people away from their weight-loss plans, but let me share a secret that you will not hear from other so-called experts:

You do not have to exercise to lose weight!

Exercise is optional, but it is highly recommended due to its many health benefits. But working out on its own is not enough to live a healthy lifestyle. Healthy eating is always the first and only required step. So, I want you to look at exercise as an added bonus and not a requirement. That mindset will create realistic expectations on your part so that if you happen to miss a day of exercise, then you won't completely give up like so many others.

Weight-loss only requires you to create a calorie deficit, so you can choose any method you want as long as you are accomplishing that goal.

You cannot out-exercise a bad diet!

The Practical Dash Diet

Consumption plays the biggest role in creating a calorie deficit. There are also other factors involved, including stress, sleep habits, and lifestyle choices. The truth is that the journey to a healthier lifestyle is a personal one that does not look the same for every person. What worked for those Internet "experts" might not work for you, and that's okay. So rather than allowing them to rip up your hopes and dreams, find your own path.

Keeping all of that in mind, exercise comes with a ton of benefits that will help you live a more productive life. So now that we understand that exercise shouldn't be placed on some unrealistic pedestal, let's dive deeper into the subject.

➤ Food choices are more important than workout choices.

➤ Exercise should become a meaningful part of your routine.

➤ If you exercise, you have to push yourself.

➤ You must find exercises that you enjoy; otherwise, you will skip them.

So, you have the right expectations now, and we have set a lot of Internet opinions straight, so let's look at some actual workouts that you can do. While we're focusing on exercises that burn the most calories in the shortest amount of time, you are free to find other options if they fit your lifestyle better.

Interval Training

Interval training is the absolute best training method for getting into top shape. This form of exercise is designed to spike your heart rate and then allow it to come down multiple times during the same workout. An example of interval training will look something like this:

Goal: 10-Minute Walk

➤ Walk for 90 seconds.

➤ Run as fast as you can for 30 seconds.

➤ Walk for 90 seconds.

➤ Run as fast as you can for 30 seconds.

➤ Walk for 90 seconds.

➤ Run as fast as you can for 30 seconds.

➤ Walk for 90 seconds.

➤ Run as fast as you can for 30 seconds.

➤ Walk for 90 seconds.

➤ Run as fast as you can for 30 seconds.

Basically, you are going all-in for a short period of time and following it with an active rest. You can use this method for all of your exercise routines. Although it's not required, it will boost the efficiency of any workout. It's easily translated into indoor cycling, treadmill workouts, and weight training.

Weight Training is the King of All Weight-Loss Workouts

There is no better workout for weight-loss than resistance training, whether you're using weights or bands. Building muscle mass is the fastest way to lower fat volume. Weight training even boosts your idle metabolic rate, which means you continue to burn calories for hours after the workout. Additionally, the higher your muscle mass, the more calories you burn throughout the day. You can also go for longer with every workout, so you'll burn even more calories. Weight training has a snowball effect in that its calorie burning potential increases exponentially as you build more muscle mass.

If this sounds like a path you want to explore, consider combining weight training with interval training. Then try creating a schedule that includes at least three sessions per week. Remember that if you miss a workout, then it's not the end of the world, so never give up.

Running

Cardio workouts are also a great choice for adding to your new lifestyle and weight-loss efforts. However, you cannot get lackadaisical here if you want to lose weight. That won't cut it. You need to include interval training here and pump up that heart rate! Better yet, set up that incline on your treadmill. Running uphill forces you to work your legs even more, leading to increased metabolism.

Running workouts are best done in the morning. While this rule is not set in stone, cardio workouts create an oxygen deficit in your body which means that it will have to work throughout the day to make up for the loss. As a result, your metabolic rate will be significantly boosted.

If running is not your cup of tea, then you can try swimming instead. Of course, you will need access to a pool, so it's not exactly the most convenient form of exercise, but it is actually more efficient that running. Maybe mix up your cardio workouts by adding the occasional swimming routine?

Train Like a Boxer

At its core, boxing is just a form of interval training, but hitting a punching bag is an amazing form of stress relief. Just make sure you do it right. Beginners often use their arm strength to throw punches, but that's a mistake. The majority of punches should come from the core, using muscles that almost every other workout ignores.

Boxers often incorporate trainers to help them keep their intensity up, but you can find a few smartphone apps to help. Just make sure that you look up proper techniques so that you are getting the most from the exercise.

The Practical Dash Diet

Jumping Rope

Kick it back to those old P.E. days, and break out the jump rope for an amazingly effective cardio workout. This is a cheap and portable tool, but more importantly, it's a lot of fun. It only takes a few minutes to get your heart racing. You probably won't want to jump rope every day, but you can use it periodically to add enjoyment to your workouts. Here's a quick and easy routine:

1. Do light rope skips for a minute to warm up?
2. Do 50 traditional jumps.
3. Follow up with 10 sprint jumps running as fast as you can.
4. Repeat Step 2 and Step 3 for 10 minutes.

Again, it's important to remember that exercise is not set in stone. The only thing that's necessary for the DASH diet is to eat healthy, so don't put exercise on such a high pedestal that it becomes intimidating. Exercise is a powerful supporting mechanic of the DASH, diet but it's not the primary tool.

Making DASH Work For You:

Now comes the time when you can begin to make your plans for using the DASH diet to meet your own personal goals. The biggest first step is to understand precisely what those goals might be.

For example, people who use the DASH diet might be:

- Attempting to control blood pressure through diet rather than medication;
- Seeking to transition themselves (and their family) into a healthier way of life;
- Trying to lose weight;
- Hoping to develop a plan for eating that is simple and which can be used throughout life instead of temporarily to address a health issue; or
- All of these things.

So, ask yourself why you are exploring the DASH diet and if you can get more than just a single result from your efforts. This matters because we are going to encourage you to make plans and track results to prove to yourself that your hard work is really paying off.

Consider that you might be doing the DASH diet only to control blood pressure. If that is the case, you need to begin finding ways to measure the blood pressure on a fairly regular basis, keep track of the figures, and talk with a physician to be sure you are remaining healthy.

Are You Trying Losing Weight or Manage Your Blood Pressure?

That is the most common question that many people ask themselves. While there are all kinds of insurance tables and expert opinions about weight, it is really a matter of your personal opinion. You could be a very large framed person of average height and read that your weight falls into an "overweight" category, but that might be incredibly inaccurate. The same applies for the small framed person with a petite build who reads that they are underweight when they are, in fact, extremely healthy.

So, the best way to understand if you are in a healthy weight range is to speak directly with your physician. They will measure body weight, height, the amount of body fat you carry, and any other factors that indicate whether you should drop weight, gain weight, or maintain your current weight.

The good news is that the DASH diet can meet all three needs because it can be designed to accommodate calorie counts as well as sodium intake levels!

After asking a physician for an expert opinion about your weight, it is time to discover the number of calories you require to maintain your current weight. This is known as the Basal Metabolic Rate, or the BMR.

The BMR

The BMR is basically the amount of energy required to allow your body to function "at rest". This means that the BMR measures the number of calories you NEED each day to maintain your current weight, and also figures this number based on ZERO energy expenditure. In other words - your BMR is the number of calories you could eat

The Practical Dash Diet

during a single day if all you did was lie on the couch.

Interestingly enough, however, you use around 60 to 70 percent of your daily calories in this way-just functioning without activity. You also burn around 10% of the calories you use when digesting as well. Yes, you can calculate ten percent of the daily calorie intake and subtract it because your body uses energy to extract energy!

How do you know your BMR? Use the "Harris Benedict" formulas below:

Adult female: 655 + (4.3 x weight in lbs.) + (4.7 x height in inches) - (4.7 x age in years); or

Adult male: 66 + (6.3 x body weight in lbs.) + (12.9 x height in inches) - (6.8 x age in years).

Here is an example of a 42-year-old woman who stands 5'7" and weighs 145 pounds.

655 + 623.5 + 314.9 - 197.4 = 1396 calories per day and fully at rest

When you have that number you also know the type of diet you must consume each day if you are trying to lose weight, gain weight, or simply maintain your weight. Now, before you argue that the woman described above would have to seriously restrict calorie intake to drop weight, remember that the figure is for a body at total rest.

If you add 30 minutes of activity each day, you also alter the number of calories that have to be consumed to maintain the weight as well. For example, if that woman took a brisk 45 minute walk each day, did regular house chores, and played with her kids for an hour, it would bump up the number of calories she could consume without gaining weight.

Take a few moments to calculate your BMR and jot it down. Then consider what your goals might be: lose weight, gain weight, or maintain current weight.

- If you are seeking to lose weight you should try to lose no more than two pounds each week - which is seven thousand calories subtracted from the diet! To do this would mean to create a daily deficit in the BMR. The woman described above would have to monitor food intake, track calories, and really boost her activity level tremendously to drop that much weight in a single week. Thus, it is best to lose weight in increments like half of a pound to a pound per week.
- To gain weight is just the reverse. The dieter would choose a higher calorie eating plan and do only enough exercise for health rather than for calorie burning. In other words, they could use the 2000 or 2600 calorie eating plan and do around 30 minutes to an hour of exercise each day and slowly gain weight.
- The person seeking to maintain their weight need only calculate the BMR and use an eating plan and exercise regimen that kept their daily calories at the BMR amount determined.
- After you understand caloric needs, it is much easier to begin using DASH for your chosen goals.

No matter what you do, the DASH diet is going to drop your sodium intake, which tends to release fluid held in the body - often called "water weight" - and that can feel like weight loss. If you stick with the diet, that water weight will stay away too!

Of course, the DASH plan is remarkably helpful in this way because it is richer in potassium than many other diets. This is a natural compound that is great for keeping

The Practical Dash Diet

blood pressure at health levels. The National Institutes for Health reported that a potassium rich diet did reduce higher blood pressures, but also insisted that it was food sources and not supplements that generated the best results.

They recommended that fish, dairy, and fruits and vegetables be put to use as the primary sources because of their bioavailable potassium that helps with bone loss and other issues.

So, not only is reducing the sodium in your diet part of the DASH plan but adding nutrients that also help to regulate blood pressure and metabolism is as well.

Getting Started with The DASH Diet

How exactly does one begin "doing" the DASH diet? It is all a matter of tracking the foods eaten and making sure to stay within the established guidelines. You are going to have to choose if you are going for the standard sodium level of 2300mg or if you are doing it for optimal reduction in the blood pressure and consuming no more than 1500 mg per day.

Either way, the DASH eating plan looks like this:

- Total fat: 27% of calories
- Saturated fat: 6% of calories
- Protein: 18% of calories
- Carbohydrate: 55% of calories
- Fiber: 30 g
- Cholesterol: 150 mg
- Sodium: 1,500 to 2,300 mg
- Potassium: 4,700 mg
- Calcium: 1,250 mg
- Magnesium: 500 mg

As you can see, the diet is very heart healthy and limits cholesterol and saturated fats to minimal amounts. The boost in nutrients, protein, and fiber are also extremely healthy, but it is the sodium where the biggest returns can be found.

Some Words on Sodium

The DASH diet tries to avoid heavy use of low sodium or specialty products. Instead, it asks you to remember that your food choices are what impact your results and success levels the most. In fact, the NIH emphasized that only a small amount of the sodium consumed each day comes from a salt shaker on the table. Instead, they report that it is processed food that is to blame for the SAD's high sodium intake.

The Practical Dash Diet

They recommend label reading and the purchase of "low sodium" labeled foods as some of the best ways to control this hidden sodium intake. For example, baked goods, seasonings, soy sauces, and even some OTC antacids are extremely high in dietary sodium according to their reports.

It helps to visualize your daily limits in order to understand how your choices play such a dramatic role in the outcome. Those using the 2,300 mg plan should imagine a teaspoon measure of table salt as their daily "cap". Those on the heavily restricted sodium plans, the 1,500 mg diets, should imagine 2/3 of a teaspoon as their daily limit.

That is not a lot at all, but many restaurant and pre-packaged foods have far more than these daily limits. Consider this list of common DASH foods and the amount of sodium they contain:

Low fat and fat free dairy products

- o   Milk, 1 cup: 107mg

- o   Yogurt, 1 cup: 175mg

- o   Cheese, 1.5 ounces: up to 450 mg

Whole grain products

- o   Cooked rice, pasta, or cereal, 1/2 cup: 5mg

- o   Bread, 1 slice: 175mg

Lean meats

- o   Canned tuna, 3 ounces: 350mg

- o   Fresh meat, poultry or fish, 3 ounces: 90mg

You could eat a large amount of these healthy foods without worrying greatly about the sodium content. If, on the other hand, you opted for a slice of roasted ham (1020mg), a glass of tomato juice (330mg), and a 1/2 of canned beans (400mg), you could easily exceed your daily amounts quickly.

Thus, the DASH dieter has to start thinking in terms of "whole foods" rather than any sort of processed, pre-cooked, or pre-packaged foods, and has to transition themselves into a diet that is flavored with herbs and citrus rather than salt and bottled sau

The Practical Dash Diet

Dash Recipe Box:

Easy Veggie Muffins

Preparation time: **10 minutes**

Cooking time: **40 minutes**

Servings: **4**

Ingredients:
¾ cup cheddar cheese, shredded
1 cup green onion, chopped
1 cup tomatoes, chopped
1 cup broccoli, chopped
2 cups non-fat milk
1 cup whole wheat biscuit mix
4 eggs
Cooking spray
1 teaspoon Italian seasoning
A pinch of black pepper

Directions:
1.   Grease a muffin tray with cooking spray and divide broccoli, tomatoes cheese and onions in each muffin cup.
2.   In a bowl, combine green onions with milk, biscuit mix, eggs, pepper and Italian seasoning, whisk well and pour into the muffin tray as well.
3.   Cook the muffins in the oven at 375 degrees F for 40 minutes, divide them between plates and serve.
Enjoy!

Nutrition Facts	
Servings: 4	
Amount per serving	
Calories	222
	% Daily Value*
Total Fat 12.1g	**16%**

The Practical Dash Diet

Nutrition Facts

Servings: 4

Saturated Fat 5.9g	**30%**
Cholesterol 189mg	**63%**
Sodium 272mg	**12%**
Total Carbohydrate 11.9g	**4%**
Dietary Fiber 1.8g	**6%**
Total Sugars 8.7g	
Protein 16.3g	

Carrot Muffins

Preparation time: **10 minutes**

Cooking time: **30 minutes**

Servings: **5**

Ingredients:
1 and ½ cups whole wheat flour
½ cup stevia
1 teaspoon baking powder
½ teaspoon cinnamon powder
½ teaspoon baking soda
¼ cup natural apple juice
¼ cup olive oil
1 egg
1 cup fresh cranberries
2 carrots, grated
2 teaspoons ginger, grated
¼ cup pecans, chopped
Cooking spray

Directions:
1.   In a large bowl, combine the flour with the stevia, baking powder, cinnamon and baking soda and stir well.

2.   Add apple juice, oil, egg, cranberries, carrots, ginger and pecans and stir really well.

3.   Grease a muffin tray with cooking spray, divide the muffin mix, introduce in the oven and cook at 375 degrees F for 30 minutes.

4.   Divide the muffins between plates and serve for breakfast. Enjoy!

Nutrition Facts	
Servings: 5	
Amount per serving	
Calories	263
	% Daily Value*
Total Fat 11.6g	15%
Saturated Fat 1.8g	9%
Cholesterol 33mg	11%
Sodium 157mg	7%
Total Carbohydrate 34.1g	12%
Dietary Fiber 2.5g	9%
Total Sugars 2.2g	
Protein 5.3g	

Pineapple Oatmeal

Preparation time: **10 minutes**

Cooking time: **25 minutes**

Servings: **4**

Ingredients:
2 cups old-fashioned oats
1 cup walnuts, chopped
2 cups pineapple, cubed
1 tablespoon ginger, grated
2 cups non-fat milk
2 eggs

2 tablespoons stevia
2 teaspoons vanilla extract

Directions:

1. In a bowl, combine the oats with the pineapple, walnuts and ginger, stir and divide into 4 ramekins.

2. In a bowl, combine the milk with the eggs, stevia and vanilla, whisk well and pour over the oats mix.

3. Introduce in the oven and cook at 400 degrees F for 25 minutes.

4. Serve for breakfast.

Enjoy!

Nutrition Facts	
Servings: 4	
Amount per serving	
Calories	471
	% Daily Value*
Total Fat 23.4g	30%
Saturated Fat 2.2g	11%
Cholesterol 84mg	28%
Sodium 100mg	4%
Total Carbohydrate 48.3g	18%
Dietary Fiber 7.5g	27%
Total Sugars 15.4g	
Protein 20.1g	

Spinach Muffins

Preparation time: **10 minutes**

Cooking time: **30 minutes**

Servings: **6**

Ingredients:

6 eggs
½ cup non-fat milk
1 cup low-fat cheese, crumbled
4 ounces spinach
½ cup roasted red pepper, chopped
2 ounces prosciutto, chopped
Cooking spray

Directions:
1. In a bowl, combine the eggs with the milk, cheese, spinach, red pepper and prosciutto and whisk well.
2. Grease a muffin tray with cooking spray, divide the muffin mix, introduce in the oven and bake at 350 degrees F for 30 minutes.
3. Divide between plates and serve for breakfast.
Enjoy!

Nutrition Facts	
Servings: 6	
Amount per serving	
Calories	168
	% Daily Value*
Total Fat 11.2g	14%
Saturated Fat 5.5g	28%
Cholesterol 189mg	63%
Sodium 354mg	15%
Total Carbohydrate 3.4g	1%
Dietary Fiber 0.6g	2%
Total Sugars 2.2g	
Protein 13.6g	

Chia Seeds Breakfast Mix

Preparation time: **8 hours**

Cooking time: **0 minutes**

Servings: **4**

Ingredients:
2 cups old-fashioned oats
4 tablespoons chia seeds
4 tablespoons coconut sugar
3 cups coconut milk
1 teaspoon lemon zest, grated
1 cup blueberries

Directions:
1.   In a bowl, combine the oats with chia seeds, sugar, milk, lemon zest and blueberries, stir, divide into cups and keep in the fridge for 8 hours.
2.   Serve for breakfast.
Enjoy!

Nutrition Facts	
Servings: 4	
Amount per serving	
Calories	681
	% Daily Value*
Total Fat 45.7g	59%
Saturated Fat 38.5g	193%
Cholesterol 0mg	0%
Sodium 69mg	3%
Total Carbohydrate 61.4g	22%
Dietary Fiber 9g	32%
Total Sugars 10g	
Protein 10.7g	
Vitamin D 0mcg	0%
Calcium 52mg	4%
Iron 5mg	29%

The Practical Dash Diet

Nutrition Facts

Servings: 4

Potassium 649mg   14%

Breakfast Fruits Bowls

Preparation time: **10 minutes**

Cooking time: **0 minutes**

Servings: **2**

Ingredients:
1 cup mango, chopped
1 banana, sliced
1 cup pineapple, chopped
1 cup almond milk

Directions:
1.   In a bowl, combine the mango with the banana, pineapple and almond milk, stir, divide into smaller bowls and serve for breakfast.
Enjoy!

Nutrition Facts

Servings: 2

Amount per serving	
Calories	419
	% Daily Value*
Total Fat 29.2g	37%
Saturated Fat 25.5g	128%
Cholesterol 0mg	0%
Sodium 20mg	1%
Total Carbohydrate 43.3g	16%

Dietary Fiber 6.6g	24%
Total Sugars 30.6g	
Protein 4.5g	

Pumpkin Breakfast Cookies

Preparation time: **10 minutes**

Cooking time: **25 minutes**

Servings: **6**

Ingredients:
2 cups whole wheat flour
1 cup old-fashioned oats
1 teaspoon baking soda
1 teaspoon pumpkin pie spice
15 ounces pumpkin puree
1 cup coconut oil, melted
1 cup coconut sugar
1 egg
½ cup pepitas, roasted
½ cup cherries, dried

Directions:
1.   In a bowl, combine the flour with the oats, baking soda, pumpkin spice, pumpkin puree, oil, sugar, egg, pepitas and cherries, stir well, shape medium cookies out of this mix, arrange them all on a lined baking sheet, introduce in the oven and bake at 350 degrees F for 25 minutes.
2.   Serve the cookies for breakfast.
Enjoy!

Nutrition Facts	
Servings: 6	
Amount per serving	
Calories	**633**
	% Daily Value*
Total Fat 43.6g	**56%**

The Practical Dash Diet

Nutrition Facts	
Servings: 6	
Saturated Fat 33.5g	168%
Cholesterol 27mg	9%
Sodium 323mg	14%
Total Carbohydrate 51.3g	19%
Dietary Fiber 5.6g	20%
Total Sugars 3g	
Protein 11.3g	

Delicious Veggie Quesadillas

Preparation time: **10 minutes**

Cooking time: **4 minutes**

Servings: **3**

Ingredients:
1 cup black beans, cooked
½ red bell pepper, chopped
4 tablespoons cilantro, chopped
½ cup corn
1 cup low-fat cheddar, shredded
6 whole wheat tortillas
1 carrot, shredded
1 small jalapeno pepper, chopped
1 cup non-fat yogurt
Juice of ½ lime

Directions:
1.   Divide black beans, red bell pepper, 2 tablespoons cilantro, corn, carrot, jalapeno and the cheese on half of the tortillas and cover with the other ones.
2.   Heat up a pan over medium-high heat, add one quesadilla, cook for 3 minutes on one side, flip, cook for 1 more minute on the other and transfer to a plate.
3.   Repeat with the rest of the quesadillas.
4.   In a bowl, combine 2 tablespoons cilantro with yogurt and lime juice, whisk well and serve next to the quesadillas

Enjoy!

Nutrition Facts	
Servings: 3	
Amount per serving	
Calories	479
	% Daily Value*
Total Fat 3.3g	4%
Saturated Fat 0.3g	2%
Cholesterol 0mg	0%
Sodium 285mg	12%
Total Carbohydrate 92.8g	34%
Dietary Fiber 17.4g	62%
Total Sugars 4.3g	
Protein 23.3g	

Chicken Wraps

Preparation time: **10 minutes**

Cooking time: **10 minutes**

Servings: **4**

Ingredients:
8 ounces chicken breast, cubed
½ cup celery, chopped
2/3 cup mandarin oranges, chopped
¼ cup onion, chopped
A drizzle of olive oil
2 tablespoons mayonnaise
¼ teaspoon garlic powder

A pinch of black pepper
4 whole wheat tortillas
4 lettuce leaves

Directions:
1.   Heat up a pan with the oil over medium-high heat, add chicken cubes, cook for 5 minutes on each side and transfer to a bowl.
2.   Divide the chicken on each tortilla, also divide celery, oranges, onion, mayo, garlic powder, black pepper and lettuce leaves, wrap and serve for lunch.
Enjoy!

Nutrition Facts	
Servings: 4	
Amount per serving	
Calories	240
	% Daily Value*
Total Fat 5.5g	7%
Saturated Fat 0.5g	2%
Cholesterol 38mg	13%
Sodium 224mg	10%
Total Carbohydrate 30.8g	11%
Dietary Fiber 4.4g	16%
Total Sugars 6g	
Protein 17g	
Vitamin D 0mcg	0%
Calcium 55mg	4%
Iron 2mg	9%
Potassium 318mg	7%

Black Bean Patties

Preparation time: **10 minutes**

Cooking time: **10 minutes**

Servings: **4**

Ingredients:
2 whole wheat bread slices, torn
3 tablespoons cilantro, chopped
2 garlic cloves, minced
15 ounces canned black beans, no-salt-added, drained and rinsed
6 ounces canned chipotle peppers, chopped
1 teaspoon cumin, ground
1 egg
Cooking spray
½ avocado, peeled, pitted and mashed
1 tablespoon lime juice
1 cherry tomato, chopped

Directions:
1.   Put the bread in your food processor, pulse well and transfer bread crumbs to a bowl.
2.   Combine them with cilantro, garlic, black beans, chipotle peppers, cumin and egg, stir well and shape 4 patties out of this mix.
3.   Heat up a pan over medium-high heat, grease with cooking spray, add beans patties, cook them for 5 minutes on each side and transfer to plates.
4.   In a bowl, combine the avocado with tomato and lime juice, stir well, add over the patties and serve for lunch.
        Enjoy!

Nutrition Facts	
Servings: 4	
Amount per serving	
Calories	487
	% Daily Value*
Total Fat 8.3g	11%
Saturated Fat 1.9g	10%
Cholesterol 41mg	14%

The Practical Dash Diet

Sodium 93mg	**4%**
Total Carbohydrate 79.1g	**29%**
Dietary Fiber 19.5g	**70%**
Total Sugars 5.5g	
Protein 27.7g	

Lunch Rice Bowls

Preparation time: **10 minutes**

Cooking time: **5 minutes**

Servings: **2**

Ingredients:
1 teaspoon olive oil
1 cup mixed bell peppers, onion, zucchini and corn, chopped
1 cup chicken meat, cooked and shredded
1 cup brown rice, cooked
3 tablespoons salsa
2 tablespoons low-fat cheddar, shredded
2 tablespoons low-fat sour cream

Directions:
1.   Heat up a pan with the oil over medium-high heat, add mixed veggies, stir and cook them for 5 minutes.
2.   Divide the rice and the chicken meat into 2 bowls, add mixed veggies and top each with salsa, cheese and sour cream.
3.   Serve for lunch.
Enjoy!

Nutrition Facts	
Servings: 2	
Amount per serving	
Calories	**540**
	% Daily Value*
Total Fat 12.8g	**16%**

Nutrition Facts	
Servings: 2	
Saturated Fat 3.9g	**20%**
Cholesterol 68mg	**23%**
Sodium 224mg	**10%**
Total Carbohydrate 76.3g	**28%**
Dietary Fiber 4.2g	**15%**
Total Sugars 1.7g	
Protein 28.9g	
Vitamin D 0mcg	0%
Calcium 78mg	6%
Iron 3mg	16%
Potassium 661mg	14%

Salmon Sandwich

Preparation time: **10 minutes**

Cooking time: **0 minutes**

Servings: **3**

Ingredients:
1 cup canned salmon, flaked
1 tablespoon lemon juice
3 tablespoons fat-free yogurt
2 tablespoons red bell pepper, chopped
1 teaspoon capers, drained and chopped
1 tablespoon red onion, chopped
1 teaspoon dill, chopped
A pinch of black pepper
3 whole wheat bread slices

Directions:
1.   In a bowl, combine the salmon with the lemon juice, yogurt, bell pepper, capers, onion, dill and black pepper and stir well.

The Practical Dash Diet

2.   Spread this on each bread slice and serve for lunch. Enjoy!

Nutrition Facts	
Servings: 3	
Amount per serving	
Calories	**107**
	% Daily Value*
Total Fat 1.3g	**2%**
Saturated Fat 0.3g	**1%**
Cholesterol 0mg	**0%**
Sodium 176mg	**8%**
Total Carbohydrate 19.4g	**7%**
Dietary Fiber 3.1g	**11%**
Total Sugars 7g	
Protein 5.5g	
Vitamin D 0mcg	0%
Calcium 75mg	6%
Iron 1mg	7%
Potassium 282mg	6%

Stuffed Mushrooms Caps

Preparation time: **10 minutes**

Cooking time: **15 minutes**

Servings: **2**

Ingredients:
2 Portobello mushroom caps
2 tablespoons pesto
2 tomato, chopped
¼ cup low-fat mozzarella, shredded

Directions:
1.   Divide pesto, tomato and mozzarella in each mushroom cap, arrange them on a lined baking sheet, introduce in the oven and bake at 400 degrees F for 15 minutes.
2.   Serve for lunch.
Enjoy!

Nutrition Facts	
Servings: 2	
Amount per serving	
Calories	**81**
	% Daily Value*
Total Fat 6.7g	9%
Saturated Fat 1.3g	6%
Cholesterol 4mg	1%
Sodium 103mg	4%
Total Carbohydrate 3.7g	1%
Dietary Fiber 1.1g	4%
Total Sugars 2.8g	
Protein 2.5g	
Vitamin D 32mcg	162%
Calcium 59mg	5%
Iron 1mg	3%

Nutrition Facts

Servings: 2

Potassium 176mg   4%

Lunch Tuna Salad

Preparation time: **10 minutes**

Cooking time: **0 minutes**

Servings: **3**

Ingredients:
5 ounces canned tuna in water, drained
1 tablespoon red vinegar
1 tablespoon olive oil
¼ cup green onions, chopped
2 cups arugula
1 tablespoon low-fat parmesan, grated
A pinch of black pepper
2 ounces whole wheat pasta, cooked

Directions:
1.   In a bowl, combine the tuna with the vinegar, oil, green onions, arugula, pasta and black pepper and toss.

2.   Divide between 3 plates, sprinkle parmesan on top and serve for lunch.

Enjoy!

Nutrition Facts	
Servings: 3	
Amount per serving	
Calories	182
	% Daily Value*
Total Fat 7g	9%

Nutrition Facts

Servings: 3

Saturated Fat 1.3g	6%
Cholesterol 21mg	7%
Sodium 58mg	3%
Total Carbohydrate 15.1g	5%
Dietary Fiber 2.1g	8%
Total Sugars 1.1g	
Protein 14.3g	
Vitamin D 0mcg	0%
Calcium 60mg	5%
Iron 1mg	8%
Potassium 262mg	6%

Oven Roasted Herbed Carrots

Preparation time: **10 minutes**

Cooking time: **40 minutes**

Servings: **6**

Ingredients:
15 carrots, halved lengthwise
2 tablespoons coconut sugar
¼ cup olive oil
½ teaspoon rosemary, dried
½ teaspoon garlic powder
A pinch of black pepper

Directions:
1.   In a bowl, combine the carrots with the sugar, oil, rosemary, garlic powder and black pepper, toss well, spread on a lined baking sheet, introduce in the oven and bake at 400 degrees F for 40 minutes.
2.   Divide between plates and serve as a side dish.
Enjoy!

The Practical Dash Diet

Nutrition Facts	
Servings: 6	
Amount per serving	
Calories	167
	% Daily Value*
Total Fat 8.4g	11%
Saturated Fat 1.2g	6%
Cholesterol 0mg	0%
Sodium 118mg	5%
Total Carbohydrate 21.6g	8%
Dietary Fiber 3.8g	14%
Total Sugars 7.6g	
Protein 1.6g	
Vitamin D 0mcg	0%
Calcium 52mg	4%
Iron 1mg	3%
Potassium 491mg	10%

Tasty Grilled Asparagus

Preparation time: **10 minutes**

Cooking time: **6 minutes**

Servings: **4**

Ingredients:
2 pounds asparagus, trimmed
2 tablespoons olive oil
A pinch of salt and black pepper

Directions:

1.	In a bowl, combine the asparagus with salt, pepper and oil and toss well.

2.	Place the asparagus on preheated grill over medium-high heat, cook for 3 minutes on each side, divide between plates and serve as a side dish.

Enjoy!

Nutrition Facts	
Servings: 4	
Amount per serving	
Calories	**105**
	% Daily Value*
Total Fat 7.3g	**9%**
Saturated Fat 1.1g	**5%**
Cholesterol 0mg	**0%**
Sodium 5mg	**0%**
Total Carbohydrate 8.8g	**3%**
Dietary Fiber 4.8g	**17%**
Total Sugars 4.3g	
Protein 5g	
Vitamin D 0mcg	0%
Calcium 55mg	4%
Iron 5mg	27%
Potassium 459mg	10%

Easy Roasted Broccoli

Preparation time: **10 minutes**

Cooking time: **30 minutes**

Servings: **4**

Ingredients:
2 pounds Broccoli, broken down into large florets
A pinch of black pepper
3 tablespoons olive oil
2 tablespoons parsley, chopped

Directions:
1. Arrange the broccoli on a lined baking sheet, add black pepper and oil, toss, put it in the oven and cook at 400 degrees F for 30 minutes.
2. Add parsley, toss, divide between plates and serve as a side dish. Enjoy!

Nutrition Facts	
Servings: 4	
Amount per serving	
Calories	**184**
	% Daily Value*
Total Fat 10.5g	**13%**
Saturated Fat 1.5g	**8%**
Cholesterol 0mg	**0%**
Sodium 157mg	**7%**
Total Carbohydrate 22.5g	**8%**
Dietary Fiber 5.7g	**20%**
Total Sugars 11.2g	
Protein 1.9g	
Vitamin D 0mcg	0%
Calcium 77mg	6%
Iron 1mg	4%
Potassium 736mg	16%

The Practical Dash Diet

Baked Potato Mix

Preparation time: **10 minutes**

Cooking time: 1 hour and 15 minutes

Servings: **8**

Ingredients:
6 potatoes, peeled and sliced
2 garlic cloves, minced
2 tablespoons olive oil
1 and ½ cups coconut cream
¼ cup coconut milk
1 tablespoon thyme, chopped
¼ teaspoon nutmeg, ground
A pinch of red pepper flakes
1 and ½ cups low-fat cheddar, shredded
½ cup low-fat parmesan, grated

Directions:
1.   Heat up a pan with the oil over medium heat, add garlic, stir and cook for 1 minute.
2.   Add coconut cream, coconut milk, thyme, nutmeg and pepper flakes, stir, bring to a simmer, reduce heat to low and cook for 10 minutes.
3.   Arrange 1/3 of the potatoes in a baking dish, add 1/3 of the cream, repeat with the rest of the potatoes and the cream, sprinkle the cheddar on top, cover with tin foil, introduce in the oven and cook at 375 degrees F for 45 minutes.
4.   Uncover the dish, sprinkle the parmesan, bake everything for 20 minutes, divide between plates and serve as a side dish.
Enjoy!

Nutrition Facts	
Servings: 8	
Amount per serving	
Calories	**313**
	% Daily Value*
Total Fat 18.3g	**23%**
Saturated Fat 12.9g	**65%**

The Practical Dash Diet

Nutrition Facts

Servings: 8	
Cholesterol 6mg	2%
Sodium 192mg	8%
Total Carbohydrate 29.1g	11%
Dietary Fiber 5.2g	18%
Total Sugars 3.8g	
Protein 10.9g	
Vitamin D 0mcg	0%
Calcium 149mg	11%
Iron 2mg	12%
Potassium 814mg	17%

Spicy Brussels Sprouts

Preparation time: **10 minutes**

Cooking time: **20 minutes**

Servings: **6**

Ingredients:
2 pounds Brussels sprouts, halved
2 tablespoons olive oil
A pinch of black pepper
1 tablespoon sesame oil
2 garlic cloves, minced
½ cup coconut aminos
2 teaspoons apple cider vinegar
1 tablespoon coconut sugar
2 teaspoons chili sauce
A pinch of red pepper flakes
Sesame seeds for serving

Directions:

The Practical Dash Diet

1.   Spread the sprouts on a lined baking dish, add the olive oil, the sesame oil, black pepper, garlic, aminos, vinegar, coconut sugar, chili sauce and pepper flakes, toss well, introduce in the oven and bake at 425 degrees F for 20 minutes.

2.   Divide the sprouts between plates, sprinkle sesame seeds on top and serve as a side dish.

Enjoy!

Nutrition Facts	
Servings: 6	
Amount per serving	
Calories	**164**
	% Daily Value*
Total Fat 7.6g	**10%**
Saturated Fat 1.2g	**6%**
Cholesterol 0mg	**0%**
Sodium 110mg	**5%**
Total Carbohydrate 21.4g	**8%**
Dietary Fiber 5.7g	**20%**
Total Sugars 3.3g	
Protein 5.4g	
Vitamin D 0mcg	0%
Calcium 55mg	4%
Iron 2mg	11%
Potassium 597mg	13%

Easy Slow Cooked Potatoes

Preparation time: **10 minutes**

Cooking time: **6 hours**

Servings: **6**

Ingredients:
Cooking spray
2 pounds baby potatoes, quartered
3 cups low-fat cheddar cheese, shredded
2 garlic cloves, minced
8 bacon slices, cooked and chopped
¼ cup green onions, chopped
1 tablespoon sweet paprika
A pinch of black pepper

Directions:
1.   Spray a slow cooker with the cooking spray, add baby potatoes, cheddar, garlic, bacon, green onions, paprika and black pepper, toss, cover and cook on High for 6 hours.
2.   Divide between plates and serve as a side dish. Enjoy!

Nutrition Facts	
Servings: 6	
Amount per serving	
Calories	323
	% Daily Value*
Total Fat 19.1g	**25%**
Saturated Fat 12g	**60%**
Cholesterol 60mg	**20%**
Sodium 371mg	**16%**
Total Carbohydrate 20.8g	**8%**
Dietary Fiber 4.4g	**16%**
Total Sugars 0.5g	
Protein 18.3g	

The Practical Dash Diet

Nutrition Facts	
Servings: 6	
Vitamin D 7mcg	34%
Calcium 460mg	35%
Iron 6mg	31%
Potassium 724mg	15%

Squash Side Salad

Preparation time: **10 minutes**

Cooking time: **30 minutes**

Servings: **6**

Ingredients:
1 cup orange juice
3 tablespoons coconut sugar
1 and ½ tablespoons mustard
1 tablespoon ginger, grated
1 and ½ pounds butternut squash, peeled and roughly cubed
Cooking spray
A pinch of black pepper
1/3 cup olive oil
6 cups salad greens
1 radicchio, sliced
½ cup pistachios, roasted

Directions:
1.   In a bowl, combine the orange juice with the sugar, mustard, ginger, black pepper and squash, toss well, spread on a lined baking sheet, spray everything with cooking oil, introduce in the oven and bake at 400 degrees F for 30 minutes.
2.   In a salad bowl, combine the squash with salad greens, radicchio, pistachios and oil, toss well, divide between plates and serve as a side dish.
Enjoy!

Nutrition Facts

Servings: 6

Amount per serving

Calories	240

	% Daily Value*
Total Fat 14.7g	19%
Saturated Fat 2g	10%
Cholesterol 0mg	0%
Sodium 51mg	2%
Total Carbohydrate 25.6g	9%
Dietary Fiber 2.6g	9%
Total Sugars 5.7g	
Protein 3.3g	
Vitamin D 0mcg	0%
Calcium 59mg	5%
Iron 2mg	9%
Potassium 432mg	9%

Colored Iceberg Salad

Preparation time: **10 minutes**

Cooking time: **0 minutes**

Servings: **4**

Ingredients:
1 iceberg lettuce head, leaves torn
6 bacon slices, cooked and halved
2 green onions, sliced
3 carrots, shredded
6 radishes, sliced
¼ cup red vinegar

¼ cup olive oil
3 garlic cloves, minced
A pinch of black pepper

Directions:
1.   In a large salad bowl, combine the lettuce leaves with the bacon, green onions, carrots, radishes, vinegar, oil, garlic and black pepper, toss, divide between plates and serve as a side dish.
Enjoy!

Nutrition Facts	
Servings: 4	
Amount per serving	
Calories	**149**
	% Daily Value*
Total Fat 12.9g	17%
Saturated Fat 1.8g	9%
Cholesterol 0mg	0%
Sodium 47mg	2%
Total Carbohydrate 8.5g	3%
Dietary Fiber 2g	7%
Total Sugars 3.4g	
Protein 1.2g	
Vitamin D 0mcg	0%
Calcium 29mg	2%
Iron 3mg	14%
Potassium 314mg	7%

Chicken Parmesan:

Preparation time: **30 minutes**

The Practical Dash Diet

Cooking time: **30 minutes**

Servings: **4**

2 tbsp. extra virgin olive oil
1 large Spaghetti Squash
2 c. Pomodoro sauce (plain marinara)
3 cloves garlic, minced
1 large yellow onion, diced
1 1/2 tsp. dried Italian seasoning
1 tsp. dried basil
Kosher salt and fresh black pepper to taste
1/4 tsp. fennel seeds (optional)
Red pepper flakes (optional)
1 lb boneless skinless chicken breast, cut into 4 equal pieces
2 tbsp flour
1 egg
¼ c. crushed bran cereal (or low sodium breadcrumbs)
¼ c. finely grated parmesan

Instructions:

1. In a skillet over medium heat, heat the olive oil. Sauté the onions for 5 minutes, then add the garlic and cook for 2 more minutes stirring. Make sure nothing is sticking to the bottom of the pan. Add the fire roasted tomatoes, the pomodoro and all the herbs and spices. Stir until everything is incorporated and reduce heat to medium low, leave for 15 minutes with the lid propped.

2. Slice the spaghetti squash in half, and scoop out the seeds and pulp. Brush lightly with olive oil and season with salt and pepper.

3. Place cut side down on a foil lined baking sheet and bake at 400 degrees F, for 40-50 minutes or until the squash is very tender.

4. While the squash is cooking, crack the egg into a flat shallow dish and add a few tbsp. of water beating the mixture until combined. In another flat shallow dish, mix together the bread crumbs and parmesan.

5. Take the 4 chicken pieces and very lightly sift the flour over them so they're even coated. Shake off the excess. Then dredge them in the egg mixture then in the parmesan bread crumb mixture evenly coating them.

6. In a large cast iron skillet, heat the other tablespoon of olive oil. Once the oil is hot, add the bread crumb coated chicken and sear until golden on both sides (2-3 min on each side).

7. Once you've seared the chicken, place in a square baking dish and pour a scoop of the tomato sauce mixture on each chicken piece. Bake in the oven (at the same time the squash is cooking) for about 20-25 minutes or until a meat thermometer reads 165 Degrees F.

8. When the squash is done, take a fork and scrape out all the flesh. It should break down into stringy, spaghetti-like pieces.

9. In 4 dishes, distribute the spaghetti squash evenly, then top with one of the chicken breasts, and finish with the rest of the tomato sauce. Top with more parmesan if desired

Enjoy!

The Practical Dash Diet

Nutrition Facts

Servings: 4

Amount per serving

Calories	332

	% Daily Value*
Total Fat 15.9g	20%
Saturated Fat 4.5g	22%
Cholesterol 85mg	28%
Sodium 496mg	39%
Total Carbohydrate 30g	11%
Dietary Fiber 3.2g	11%
Total Sugars 7.5g	
Protein 20.9g	

Slow Cooker Turkey Sweet Potato Chili:

Preparation time: **10 minutes**

Cooking time: **0 minutes**

Servings: **6**

Ingredients:
1 lb ground turkey
1 yellow onion, diced
4 cloves garlic, minced
¼ tsp. cayenne pepper (optional)
salt and pepper
3 cups chicken stock
2 (14.5 oz cans fire roasted tomatoes)
15 oz can black beans
1 cup sweet corn, from the can
1 cup dry quinoa
1 lb sweet potato, peeled and chopped into ½ inch cubes

2 Tablespoons chili powder
1 teaspoon cumin
1/2 teaspoon salt
¼ tsp. fresh black pepper
¼ c. fresh cilantro, chopped

Directions:

1. Brown the turkey, in a large skillet on the stop, then saute the onions in the meat juices until translucent. Add the garlic and continue stirring until fragrant and until the turkey is completely cooked (no pink visible). Add in the cayenne pepper and toss in a pinch of salt and pepper. Stir

2. Pour the meat mixture into the slow cooker and add all remaining ingredients except cilantro. Stir.

3. Cook on low for 3 to 3 and ½ hours or until potatoes are very tender. Or on low for 5-6 hours. Stir in Cilantro 15 minutes before eating.

4. This one is great to throw together before leaving for work and set the timer on your slow cooker. Then you'll have a delicious meal waiting for you when you return.

Nutrition Facts	
Servings: 6	
Amount per serving	
Calories	409
	% Daily Value*
Total Fat 4.6g	6%
Saturated Fat 0.8g	4%
Cholesterol 52mg	17%
Sodium 865mg	38%
Total Carbohydrate 59.8g	22%
Dietary Fiber 11.3g	40%
Total Sugars 11.5g	
Protein 34.6g	

Fennel Side Salad

Preparation time: **10 minutes**

Cooking time: **0 minutes**

Servings: **4**

Ingredients:
2 fennel bulbs, trimmed and shaved
1 and ¼ cups zucchini, sliced
2/3 cup dill, chopped
¼ cup lemon juice
¼ cup olive oil
6 cups arugula
½ cups walnuts, chopped
1/3 cup low-fat feta cheese, crumbled

Directions:
1.   In a large bowl, combine the fennel with the zucchini, dill, lemon juice, arugula, oil, walnuts and cheese, toss, divide between plates and serve as a side dish.
Enjoy!

Nutrition Facts	
Servings: 4	
Amount per serving	
Calories	**282**
	% Daily Value*
Total Fat 22.9g	**29%**
Saturated Fat 2.5g	**13%**
Cholesterol 0mg	**0%**
Sodium 98mg	**4%**
Total Carbohydrate 17.9g	**6%**
Dietary Fiber 6.9g	**25%**
Total Sugars 2.1g	
Protein 8.4g	
Vitamin D 0mcg	0%
Calcium 268mg	21%

The Practical Dash Diet

Nutrition Facts	
Servings: 4	
Iron 6mg	33%
Potassium 1108mg	24%

Shrimp Salad with Grilled Peaches:

Preparation time: **20 minutes**

Cooking time: **10 minutes**

Servings: **4**

1 / 3 cup orange juice
3 tbsp. vinegar
½ tbsp. Dijon mustard
½ tbsp. honey
1 tablespoon fresh basil, chopped

SALAD:
Olive oil cooking spray
1 pound raw shrimp, peeled and deveined
1 / 2 teaspoon lemon-pepper seasoning
8 cups spinach
1 cup cherry tomatoes, halved
1 / 2 cup scallions, chopped
2 medium peaches, halved

Directions:

1.	Whisk together the ingredients for the dressing in a small bowl and set aside.

2.	Lightly spritz the shrimp and peaches with olive oil cooking spray and light the grill. Once the grill is very hot, arrange the shrimp either on skewers or in a grill basket and grill until completely cooked (shrimp should be pink with grill marks). Place the peach halves cut side down on the grill and grill until they have grill marks and the turned slightly tender. Slice the peach halves into 1 inch cubes.

3.	Assemble the salad by tossing the greens with the tomatoes and scallions, then portion out the shrimp and peaches on top of the salad and drizzle dressing over top.

Enjoy!

The Practical Dash Diet

Nutrition Facts	
Servings: 4	
Amount per serving	
Calories	212
	% Daily Value*
Total Fat 2.6g	3%
Saturated Fat 0.7g	3%
Cholesterol 239mg	80%
Sodium 351mg	15%
Total Carbohydrate 18.3g	7%
Dietary Fiber 3.5g	13%
Total Sugars 12.7g	
Protein 29.2g	

Corn Mix

Preparation time: **10 minutes**

Cooking time: **0 minutes**

Servings: **4**

Ingredients:
½ cup cider vinegar
¼ cup coconut sugar
A pinch of black pepper
ups corn
p red onion, chopped
cucumber, sliced
red bell pepper, chopped
erry tomatoes, halved
ns parsley, chopped
basil, chopped
alapeno, chopped
gula leaves

The Practical Dash Diet

Directions:

1.   In a large bowl, combine the corn with onion, cucumber, bell pepper, cherry tomatoes, parsley, basil, jalapeno and arugula and toss.

2.   Add vinegar, sugar and black pepper, toss well, divide between plates and serve as a side dish.

Enjoy!

Nutrition Facts	
Servings: 4	
Amount per serving	
Calories	165
	% Daily Value*
Total Fat 2g	3%
Saturated Fat 0.3g	2%
Cholesterol 0mg	0%
Sodium 34mg	1%
Total Carbohydrate 35g	13%
Dietary Fiber 5.4g	19%
Total Sugars 7.6g	
Protein 6g	
Vitamin D 0mcg	0%
Calcium 32mg	2%
Iron 5mg	26%
Potassium 617mg	13%

Mediterranean Chicken with Quinoa

Preparation time: **20 minutes**

Cooking time: **25 minutes**

Servings: **4**

The Practical Dash Diet

1 lb boneless skinless chicken breast (about 4 medium or small pieces)
1 teaspoon lemon zest
½ teaspoon salt
½ teaspoon ground pepper, divided
¾ cup Quinoa
2 cups baby spinach
1 cup chopped cucumber
1 cup chopped tomato
¼ cup chopped red onion
¼ cup crumbled feta cheese
2 tablespoons lemon juice
3 tablespoons extra-virgin olive oil
½ tsp garlic powder
½ tsp dried Italian Seasoning

Directions:

1.   Brush the chicken with olive oil and season with HALF of the salt and pepper and all of the lemon zest. Bake on a baking dish at 425 degrees for about 25 minutes or until the chicken reads 165 degrees with the meat thermometer.

2.   Cook the Quinoa According to Package directions, and then as soon as it's finished cooking, stir in the fresh spinach so that it wilts slightly.

3.   Drain off any excess liquid from the quinoa and stir in the tomatoes, cucumber, onions and feta. Portion out the quinoa mixture onto each plate and top with a piece of the chicken breast.

4.   Whisk together the oil, lemon juice, garlic powder and Italian seasoning and drizzle over the dish evenly portioning out for each dish.

Enjoy!

Nutrition Facts	
Servings: 4	
Amount per serving	
Calories	472
	% Daily Value*
Total Fat 23.3g	30%
Saturated Fat 5.6g	28%
Cholesterol 110mg	37%
Sodium 511mg	22%
Total Carbohydrate 25.5g	9%
Dietary Fiber 3.5g	13%
Total Sugars 2.7g	

The Practical Dash Diet

Nutrition Facts

Servings: 4

Protein 39.9g

Persimmon Side Salad

Preparation time: **10 minutes**

Cooking time: **0 minutes**

Servings: **4**

Ingredients:
Seeds from 1 pomegranate
2 persimmons, cored and sliced
5 cups baby arugula
6 tablespoons green onions, chopped
4 navel oranges, peeled and cut into segments
¼ cup white vinegar
1/3 cup olive oil
3 tablespoons pine nuts
1 and ½ teaspoons orange zest, grated
2 tablespoons orange juice
1 tablespoon coconut sugar
½ shallot, chopped
A pinch of cinnamon powder

Directions:
1.   In a salad bowl, combine the pomegranate seeds with persimmons, arugula, green onions and oranges and toss.
2.   In another bowl, combine the vinegar with the oil, pine nuts, orange zest, orange juice, sugar, shallot and cinnamon, whisk well, add to the salad, toss and serve as a side dish.
        Enjoy!

Nutrition Facts

Servings: 4

Amount per serving

The Practical Dash Diet

Nutrition Facts

Servings: 4

Calories	**355**

	% **Daily Value***
Total Fat 21.7g	28%
Saturated Fat 2.8g	14%
Cholesterol 0mg	0%
Sodium 19mg	1%
Total Carbohydrate 40.2g	15%
Dietary Fiber 5.7g	20%
Total Sugars 21.9g	
Protein 4.1g	
Vitamin D 0mcg	0%
Calcium 127mg	10%
Iron 2mg	9%
Potassium 557mg	12%

The Practical Dash Diet

14 Day Dash Meal Plan:

The following is a 14-day sample meal plan you can use to give you an idea of how you should be eating while on the DASH diet plan. This is simply meant to help guide you and ease you into starting the nutrition plan. It's not to be used as a crutch.

Recall the phrase, "if you give a man a fish, you feed him for a day. If you teach a man to fish, you feed him for life." It wouldn't be practical for me to tell you exactly how to eat each and every day. If I tried to do that, you would end up failing because if you truly want to achieve success with this diet, you have to make it your own.

You wouldn't be able to adapt to different situations you'd find yourself in. For example, let's say you're at an office party, and you're not able to eat exactly what the meal plan laid out for you. What do you do? You'd likely freeze up because you don't know how to adapt yourself to the given situation.

On the other hand, if you know all of the ins and outs of the DASH diet (which you should by now), then you'll know what you are and aren't allowed to eat at the office party. You'll still be able to enjoy yourself without having to constantly worry if you broke your diet plan or not. With that being said, this sample meal plan is based on a 2,000 calorie a day diet. Be sure to adjust the serving and portion sizes accordingly to fit your caloric needs.

Note: You can break up these meal plan ideas into smaller meals with snacks if you like. I made the meal plans with just breakfast, lunch, and dinner, but you can modify it to have snacks if that's how you like to eat.

For example, let's say for breakfast you're going to eat 1 cup of oatmeal, 1 cup of skim milk, ½ cup of raspberries, and 1 medium banana. You could skip out on eating the banana as part of your breakfast and instead eat it a couple of hours later as a snack. It can be done either way because it works out to the same amount of calories in the end. Choose whatever works best for you and how it is that you prefer to eat.

Additionally, replace certain foods as necessary. For example, if a meal calls for ½ cup of blueberries and you like raspberries more, then go ahead and eat ½ cup of raspberries instead of blueberries. Or if you like cauliflower more than carrots, then go ahead and replace the carrots with cauliflower.

Yes, variety is good, but don't feel like you have to eat a certain fruit or vegetable that you hate when you could easily replace it with something else. Do what works best for you and will allow you to stick to this diet for a long time to come.

Finally, I didn't include any of the sweets in the meal plan. Feel free to add in whatever sweets you like throughout the week up to your allotted number of servings.

Day 1:

The Practical Dash Diet

Breakfast

- 2 Slices of Whole Wheat Toast
- 2 Tablespoons of Natural Peanut Butter (one tbsp. per slice of toast)
- 1 Medium Apple
- ½ Cup of Your Choice of Berries

Lunch

- 3 Ounces of Lean Turkey
- 1 Cup of Broccoli
- 1 Cup of Quinoa
- 1.5 Ounces of Low-Fat Yogurt

Dinner

- 3 ounces of grilled chicken
- ½ Cup of Steamed Cauliflower
- ½ Cup of Steamed Bell Peppers
- 1 Cup of Brown Rice
- 1 Medium Orange

Day 2:

Breakfast:

- 2 Scrambled Eggs
- ½ of a Whole-Wheat Pita Pocket
- ½ of a Medium Grapefruit

Lunch:

- 3 Ounces of Cod
- 2 Teaspoons of Olive Oil
- ½ Cup of Mixed Berries
- 1 Cup of Steamed Broccoli
- 1 Whole-Wheat Roll

Dinner:

- 2 Cups of Whole-Wheat Spaghetti Noodles
- ½ Cup of Grated Parmesan Cheese
- ½ Cup of Tomato Sauce
- 2 Ounces of Lean Beef

The Practical Dash Diet

Day 3:

Breakfast:

- 1 Cup of Oatmeal
- ½ Cup of Raspberries
- 1 Cup of Skim Milk
- 1 Medium Banana

Lunch:

Salad Consisting of the Following:

- 3 Ounces of Lean Grilled Chicken
- 3 Cups of Leafy Green Vegetables
- ½ Cup of Cumcumber
- ½ Tablespoon of Flax Seeds

On the Side:

- ½ Slice of Toast

Dinner:

- 1 Cup of Roasted Potatoes
- 3 Ounces of Roast Beef
- ½ Cup of Roasted Carrots
- ½ Cup of Roasted Onions

Day 4:

Breakfast:

- 3 Hard Boiled Eggs
- 2 Slices of Turkey Bacon
- 6 Ounces of Freshly Squeezed Orange Juice
- 6 Ounces of Low-Fat Yogurt

Lunch:

Sandwich Consisting of the Following:

- 2 Slices of Whole-Wheat Bread

The Practical Dash Diet

- 3 Ounces of Packaged Tuna
- 1 Tablespoon of Mayonnaise

On the Side:

- ½ Cup of Kale
- ½ Cup of Tomatoes
- ½ Cup of Spinach
- ½ Cup of Pineapple

Dinner:

- 3 Ounces of Lean Venison
- 1 Cup of Sweet Potatoes
- ½ Cup of Roasted Carrots
- ½ Cup of Roasted Bell Pepper

Day 5:

Breakfast:

Breakfast Sandwich Consisting of the Following:

- 2 Slices of Whole Wheat Toast
- 3 Slices of Turkey Bacon
- 1 Fried Egg

On the side:

- 1 Medium Apple

Lunch:

Turkey Roll-Ups Consisting of:

- 3 Ounces of Lean Turkey Meat
- 1/4 Cup of Cheese
- 2-3 Large Leaves of Romaine Lettuce
- 2 Teaspoons of Mustard

On the Side:

- 1 Medium Apple
- ½ Cup of Mixed Broccoli and Cauliflower

Dinner:

Stuffed Bell Pepper Consisting of:

- 1 Full-Sized Bell Pepper
- 1/4 Cup of Low-Fat Cheese
- ½ Cup of Chickpeas
- ¼ Cup of Dried Apricots

Day 6:

Breakfast:

- 1 Cup of Oat Bran
- 1 Cup of Skim Milk
- ½ Cup of Mixed Berries
- 6 Ounces of Freshly Squeezed Pineapple Juice

Lunch:

Sandwich Consisting of the following:

- 2 Slices of Whole-Wheat Bread
- 3 Ounces of Lean Turkey
- ¼ Cup of Low-Fat Cheese
- 2 Teaspoons of Mustard

On the side:

- 1/3 Cup of Almonds
- 1 Medium Banana
- ½ Cup of Your Choice of Vegetables

Dinner:

Fish Tacos Consisting of:

- 3 Ounces of Tilapia
- 2 Whole-Wheat Tortillas
- 1/4 Cup of Low-Fat Cheese

On the side:

The Practical Dash Diet

- 1 Medium Peach
- 1 Cup of Mixed Vegetables

Day 7:

Breakfast:

- 1 Whole-Wheat Bagel
- 2 Tablespoons of Natural Almond or Peanut Butter
- 1 Medium Pear
- 1 Cup of Skim Milk

Lunch:

Salad Consisting of the following:

- 4 Cups of Spring Mix Salad
- ¼ Cup of Severed Almonds
- ½ Cup of Orange Slices
- 2 Tablespoons of Low-Fat Dressing

Dinner:

- 3 Ounces of Salmon
- 1 Cup of Strawberries
- 1 Cup of Asparagus
- 1 Small Biscuit
- 2 Teaspoons of Olive Oil

Day 8:

Breakfast:

- 1 Cup of Oatmeal
- 1 Cup of Skim Milk
- ½ Cup of Strawberries
- ½ Cup of Mango

The Practical Dash Diet

Lunch:

Baked Potato Consisting of the Following:

- 1 Large Potato
- ¼ Cup of Shredded Cheese
- ¼ Cup of Bacon Bits
- 1 Tablespoon of Reduced Fat Sour Cream

On the side:

- 1 cup of mixed broccoli, cauliflower, and bell pepper

Dinner:

- 3 Ounces of Lean Steak
- 1 Cup of Brown Rice
- 1 Teaspoon of Olive Oil
- ½ Cup of Steamed Asparagus and Carrots

Day 9:

Breakfast:

- 2 Slices of Whole-Wheat Toast
- 2 Tablespoons of Natural Almond Butter
- 1 Medium Peach
- 1 Cup of Skim Milk

Lunch:

Salad Consisting of the Following:

- 3 Ounces of Lean Chicken
- 2 Cups of Spring Mix Salad
- 2 Tablespoons of Low-Fat Dressing
- ½ Cup of Raspberries
- 1.5 Ounces of Low-Fat Cheese

Dinner:

Stir Fry Consisting of the Following:

- 2 Cups of Snow Peas

The Practical Dash Diet

- ½ Cup of Kale
- 2 Tablespoons of Olive Oil
- 2 Cups of Quinoa
- ½ Cup of Mixed Nuts

Day 10:

Breakfast:

- 3 Scrambled Eggs
- 1 Slice of Whole-Wheat Toast
- 2 Slices of Turkey Bacon
- 6 Ounces of Yogurt
- 6 Ounces of Freshly Squeezed Orange Juice

Lunch:

Turkey and Swiss Sandwich Consisting of the Following:

- 3 Ounces of Lean Turkey
- 2 Teaspoons of Mayonnaise
- 2 Slices of a Tomato
- 1 Slice of Swiss Cheese
- 2 Slices of Whole-Wheat Bread

On the side:

½ Cup of Cauliflower and Broccoli

Dinner:

- 2 Cups of Whole-Wheat Angel Pasta
- ½ Cup of Grated Parmesan Cheese
- ½ Cup of Tomato Sauce
- 2 Ounces of Lean Venison
- 1 Cup of Mixed Vegetables

Day 11:

Breakfast:

The Practical Dash Diet

- 1 Cup of Bran Flakes Cereal
- 1 Cup of Skim Milk
- 1 Medium Apple
- 1 Slice of Whole-Wheat Toast

Lunch:

Turkey Roll-Ups Consisting of:

- 3 Ounces of Lean Turkey Meat
- 1/4 Cup of Cheddar Cheese
- 2-3 Large Leaves of Romaine Lettuce
- 2 Teaspoons of Mustard

On the Side:

- 1 Medium Pear
- ½ Cup of Mixed Brussell Sprouts

Dinner:

Fish Tacos Consisting of:

- 3 Ounces of Cod
- 2 Whole-Wheat Tortillas
- 1/4 Cup of Low-Fat Cheese

On the side:

- ½ of a Medium Grapefruit
- 1 Cup of Mixed Vegetables

Day 12:

Breakfast:

- 1 Cup of Oat Bran
- 1 Cup of Skim Milk
- 1 Medium Orange
- 1 Slice of Whole Wheat Toast
- 1 Tablespoon of Natural Peanut Butter

Lunch:

Salad Consisting of the Following:

The Practical Dash Diet

- 1 Boiled Egg
- 3 Ounces of Packaged Tuna
- 2 Cups of Leafy Green Vegetables
- ½ Cup of Diced Tomatoes
- 2 Tablespoons of Low-Fat Dressing

Dinner:

Hamburger consisting of the following:

- 3 Ounces of Lean Beef
- 1 Whole-Wheat Bun
- 1 Leaf of Romaine Lettuce
- 1 Slice of a Tomato
- 1 Slice of Cheese
- 2 Teaspoons of Mustard

On the Side:

- 1 Cup of Mixed Vegetables

Day 13:

Breakfast:

Sandwich Consisting of:

- 1 Cooked Egg
- 2 Slices of Turkey Bacon
- 2 Slices of Whole Wheat Toast
- 2 Teaspoons of Mustard
- 1 Slice of Cheese

On the side:

- 1 Medium Banana

Lunch:

Salad Consisting of the following:

- 4 Cups of Spring Mix Salad
- ¼ Cup of Severed Almonds

The Practical Dash Diet

- ½ Cup of Raspberries
- 2 Tablespoons of Low-Fat Dressing

On the side:

- 1 Whole-Wheat Roll

Dinner:

- 1 Cup of Roasted Sweet Potatoes
- 3 Ounces of Roast Beef
- ½ Cup of Roasted Bell Peppers
- ½ Cup of Roasted Onions

Day 14:

Breakfast:

- 1 Whole-Wheat Bagel
- 2 Tablespoons of Natural Almond or Peanut Butter
- 6 Ounces of Yogurt
- ½ Medium Grapefruit

Lunch:

Sandwich Consisting of:

- 3 Ounces of Lean Chicken Breast
- 2 Slices of Whole Wheat Bread
- 1 Slice of Pepper Jack Cheese
- 1 Slice of a Tomato
- 2 Teaspoons of Mayonnaise

On the Side:

- ½ Cup of Cantaloupe
- ½ Cup of Your Choice of Vegetables

Dinner:

- 3 Ounces of Salmon
- 1 Cup of Brown Rice
- 1 Cup of Cooked Spinach
- 1 Tablespoon of Mixed Nuts
1 Whole-Wheat Biscuit

The Practical Dash Diet

Shopping Lists

Vegetables—eat plenty of vegetables! Veggies are not only a great source of fiber that enables good digestion, but they are rich in vitamins and minerals that are essential to a healthy body. Choose from asparagus, beets, bell peppers, broccoli, cabbage, carrots, cauliflower, celery, corn, cucumbers, eggplant, green beans, jicama, mushrooms and leafy greens such as kale, lettuce, and spinach. You should however, limit your consumption of starchy vegetables especially during the first phase of the diet.

Whole Grains—like granola, whole grain bread, and oats. (Do not mistake whole grains with mixed grains because they are two different things.)

Fruits—avocados, apples, bananas, berries, grapefruit, grapes, lemon and lime, cantaloupe, peaches, etc. are also included in the DASH Diet list. You can consume fruits either fresh or by making smoothies out of them. Just remember to stick to the recommended servings a day.

Meat, Poultry, and Seafood—pick organic, grass-fed, or wild caught. Stick to lean meats and deli meats low in sodium. Eggs are also great source of protein, but you could also choose to use egg substitutes instead.

Herbs & Spices (dried or fresh)—skip the salt and flavor your foods with herbs and spices such as basil, oregano, thyme, rosemary, dill, bay leaf, curry, coriander, cayenne pepper, chilies, cumin, chives, parsley, garlic, onions, ginger, mint, mustard, paprika, etc.

Nuts and Seeds—choose the unsalted or raw variety of almonds, cashews, hazelnuts, sunflower seeds, and pumpkin seeds.

Beverages—Avoid sugar-laden beverages such as soda and artificially flavored juices and stick to 100% fruit juice, tea, vegetable juice, and most especially, water.

Here are the foods that you should avoid:

Trans fats—also known as "hydrogenated" or "partially hydrogenated" fats. These are unsaturated fats that have been chemically modified to increase food's shelf-life and make them solid at room temperature.

Dairy Products—derive from animals can also introduce additional saturated fat into your diet. These foods include: creams, cheeses, milk, sour cream, ice cream.

Fats and Oils—high saturated fat foods that are in this category include: butter, lard, and certain oils such as palm oil, cream-based dressings or dips.

The Practical Dash Diet

DASH Shopping List

Vegetables:

- Artichokes
- Asparagus
- Avocados
- Beets
- Bell peppers
- Broccoli
- Brussels sprouts
- Cabbage
- Carrots
- Cauliflower
- Celery
- Corn
- Cucumbers
- Eggplant
- Green beans
- Leafy greens
- Leeks
- Mushrooms
- Onions
- Peas
- Potatoes
- Radishes
- Root vegetables
- Spinach
- Squash
- Tomatoes

Fruits

- Apples
- Apricots
- Bananas
- Berries
- Cherries

The Practical Dash Diet

- Oranges
- Dates
- Figs
- Grapefruit
- Grapes
- Kiwi
- Lemons
- Limes
- Mango
- Melons
- Peaches
- Papaya
- Pears
- Pineapple
- Plums
- Prunes

Protein Sources

- Beef
- Chicken (skinless)
- Eggs
- Pork tenderloin
- Salmon
- Shrimp
- Tempeh
- Tofu
- Turkey (skinless)

Grains

- Barley
- Bran Cereal
- Brown rice
- Bulgur
- Couscous
- Kasha (buckwheat)
- Low fat granola
- Muesli
- Pasta (Whole Wheat)
- Quinoa, Millet, Amaranth
- Spelt, Triticale, Kamut
- Steel Cut Oats
- Whole Grain Cereal
- Wild rice

The Practical Dash Diet

Dairy

- Buttermilk (low fat)
- Cheese
- Cottage cheese
- Kefir
- Margarine
- Milk (low fat)
- Sour cream (low fat)
- Yogurt (low fat)

Nuts and Seeds

- Almonds
- Cashews
- Hazelnuts
- Nut butter
- Peanuts
- Pecans
- Seeds
- Soy nuts
- Walnut

Accepted Canned Goods

- Applesauce

- Beans and lentils
- Broth (low sodium)
- Chiles (diced)
- Chili sauce or hot sauce (low sodium)
- Fresh salsa or Pico de gallo (low sodium)
- Fruit-only or low-sugar spreads
- Hummus (low sodium)
- Marinara sauce (low sodium)
- Mayonnaise (low-fat)
- Mustard (low sodium)
- Oil: canola, olive, sesame
- Pesto (low sodium)
- Salad dressing (low fat)
- Salmon or tuna (in water)
- Soup (low sodium)
- Soy sauce (low sodium)
- Sun-dried tomatoes

The Practical Dash Diet

- Tomato paste (low sodium)
- Tomato sauce (low sodium)
- Tomatoes (low sodium)
- Vinegar

Helpful Extras

- Herbs (dried and fresh)

- Spices of all kinds (skip any blends that use sodium or MSG)
- Popcorn to be used in an air popper
- Dried fruits
- Herbal tea
- Sodium-free vegetable juices
- No sugar fruit juices (be sure they are 100% fruit)
- Sparkling water (a reasonable alternative to soda)

How to Read Labels

We have mentioned becoming a good label reader several times. We haven't, however, gone over what it is you must look for as you read through the labels. By now, you probably have guessed that the first thing to look at is sodium, but that is actually a bit off the mark. What you need to first consider is the serving size in the package or the can.

Why? All of the nutrient information is going to be based on that serving size. Not only does knowing how much of each package qualifies as a single serving useful in terms of planning your diet, but it also allows you to gauge whether or not a food is worth eating. For example, if a small can of beans contains more than 25% of your daily sodium, and the can is the serving size, you may not want to use it.

Remember too that any serving size is subjective, and what we eat may not actually be the recommended serving size. You may opt for a much larger "serving" or even a smaller one, and that offsets the anticipated nutrients, calories, sodium, and fat.

So, first determine an actual serving size and then checkout that sodium.

All labels have to have sodium indicated per serving size and in milligrams per serving. The labels also tell you what percentage of your daily diet the amount of sodium represents. Any food that has 5% of less of the daily value of sodium is immediately to be considered a low sodium choice. If the label shows that a food has 20% or more of the recommended sodium amount it is a high sodium food, and probably best if avoided.

What else should you know about labels? The ingredients are usually in order of greatest to least quantity. This means that if you see sodium or any sort of sodium type of compound in the first few words of the ingredients it is probably a higher sodium food.

You can then apply the details taken from a label to your daily DASH plan to understand how it fits into the equation. For instance, if you choose a can of low sodium soup as a quick lunch, you need to also check the fat it contains, double check that it is indeed a low sodium food and find out how many servings are in the can to be sure you don't overdo it when you eat it as the main component of a meal.

The Practical Dash Diet

Using the Numbers from Labels and Food Lists

You will find the information on food labels, and even on food lists that give average calorie and nutrient counts for whole foods like fruit or meat, very useful. This is because you are going to want to monitor your diet according to your written plans and be sure that everything is adding up correctly.

Remember that the daily amounts for DASH are:

- Total fat: 27% of calories
- Saturated fat: 6% of calories
- Protein: 18% of calories
- Carbohydrate: 55% of calories
- Fiber: 30 g
- Cholesterol: 150 mg
- Sodium: 1,500 to 2,300 mg
- Potassium: 4,700 mg
- Calcium: 1,250 mg
- Magnesium: 500 mg

That means you need to do a bit of math if you want to know how many of your daily calories can be comprised of the nutrients. Don't worry...we've done the math for you and provided it below.

1,600 Calorie Diets
- Total Fat: 432 of your calories can come from fat.
- Total Saturated Fat: Only 96 of those fat calories can be of the saturated kind.
- Total Carbohydrates: 880 of your daily calories can come from carbs.
- Total Protein: 288 calories should come from protein.

2,000 Calorie Diets
- Total Fat: 540 of your calories can come from fat.
- Total Saturated Fat: Only 120 of those fat calories can be of the saturated kind.
- Total Carbohydrates: 1100 of your daily calories can come from carbs.
- Total Protein: 360 calories should come from protein.

2,600 Calorie Diets
- Total Fat: 702 of your calories can come from fat.
- Total Saturated Fat: Only 156 of those fat calories can be of the saturated kind.
- Total Carbohydrates: 1430 of your daily calories can come from carbs.
- Total Protein: 468 calories should come from protein.
-

The Practical Dash Diet

With all of these figures and facts you are probably more than ready to begin planning your own DASH diet. The last chapter of Resources has the blank planners that you can use to begin tracking the way that you eat now, and then use them to develop your plans for starting to eat according to the DASH diet as well.

Conclusion

I hope this book helped you plan how to eat healthy even during busy workdays.

Many people make the mistake of neglecting the amount of salt that they are consuming and the overall effect that can have on their bodies. Salt can cause more than just fluctuations in blood pressure; it can have a large bearing on your general health.

But with the recipes mentioned in this book, you will be able to cut down on the amount of salt that you consume and also reduce your body weight.

The next step is to try these recipes, put these ideas into action and get started on a healthier lifestyle.

Thank you and good luck!

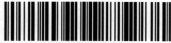

Made in the USA
Lexington, KY
16 April 2019